The Art of
Thai Foot Massage

The Art of
Thai Foot Massage

A Step by Step Guide

Simon Piers Gall

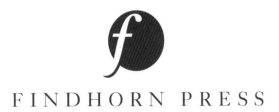

FINDHORN PRESS

First published by Findhorn Press 2008

ISBN: 978-1-84409-138-6

British Library Cataloguing-in-Publication Data.
A catalogue record for this book is available from the British Library.

Edited by Carol Shaw
Cover design by Matt Gall
Photographs by Nick ffrench
Layout by Pam Bochel
Printed and bound in the European Union

2 3 4 5 6 7 8 9 10 11 12 13 12 11 10

Published by
Findhorn Press
117-121 High Street,
Forres IV36 1AB
Scotland, UK

t +44(0)1309 690582
f +44(0)131 777 2711
e info@findhornpress.com
www.findhornpress.com

Disclaimer

Neither the publisher nor the author is engaged in rendering professional advice or services to the individual reader. The ideas, procedures, and suggestions contained in this book are not intended as a substitute for consulting with your physician. All matters regarding health require medical supervision. Neither the author nor the publisher shall be liable or responsible for any loss, injury, or damage allegedly arising from any information or suggestion in this book. The opinions expressed in this book represent the personal views of the author and not of the publisher.

Contents

Preface

I first travelled to Thailand hoping to learn a few techniques to incorporate into my existing sports massage practice. A friend had shown me a few Thai techniques that impressed me so much I immediately began to plan my trip to Thailand. This first trip was a revelation to me. Traditional Thai Massage seemed to be the perfect sports massage. The physical aspect to Thai Massage is undeniable, every joint is mobilised, every muscle is stretched and compressed in a way that has to be experienced to be appreciated, and all performed with such apparent ease by the therapist. Nearly ten years later I am still convinced that Thai Massage is the perfect sports massage; however it is also much more. As well as massaging the physical body, Traditional Thai Massage takes a holistic approach encompassing the mind, body and spirit.

As a therapist my intention was holistic, however the training I had chosen was always physical in its approach. I had begun to search for the more holistic approaches to health and well-being and was studying as a yoga teacher. I particularly enjoyed *pranayama*, or breathing techniques, and had begun incorporating *vinyasa*, combining breath with movement, into other areas of my work. Thai Massage fascinated me from the outset with its physical yet meditative approach. It combined yoga postures with massage techniques and breath work. I was immediately hooked and my interest has only increased since this first revelation. What began as a search for a few techniques to incorporate into my practice, has instead completely changed my approach, sparking an interest in all aspects of Traditional Thai Medicine, of which Thai Massage is an integral part.

After this first trip to Thailand I almost immediately returned to continue my studies. It was between these first two trips that I had my first reflexology treatment and became fascinated with the feet and also the first time I met my partner Paula. I had heard of reflexology and seen much Thai Foot Massage whilst in Thailand. I knew that it worked reflex points on the feet in order to affect the internal organs of the body, but I had never had a reflexology treatment. It wasn't that I doubted the effectiveness of the treatment, just that I preferred the physical effects of a full body massage.

Whilst waiting to return to Thailand I visited my local Complementary Therapy Centre to extol the virtues of Thai Massage and see if I could work as a therapist there. I met with the proprietor, Paula Lloyd, who was a reflexology practitioner and tutor with the ARC reflexology school. Paula seemed interested in Thai Massage and so we arranged to swap treatments. Having kept my end of the bargain I was thoroughly enjoying my reflexology treatment and fascinated by Paula's commentary throughout. The majority of the treatment was very pleasant and relaxing, except for one point where it felt like a needle was being applied to my foot. When I told Paula what I was feeling she explained that this point related to my ear. I had been experiencing constant discomfort with my ear since going scuba diving in Thailand and as I explained this to Paula, she continued to work on this area and eventually the pain died down.

After the treatment I carried on with my day thinking more about the reflexologist than the reflexology treatment. As the day wore on I noticed that when I swallowed or yawned the annoying popping sensation in my ear had subsided, and then, the next day it had gone completely, and has never recurred. After this one treatment I decided two things: to study Thai Foot Massage on my next and imminent trip to Thailand, and to get to know Paula better. I think I have managed both, as Paula and I have been together ever since and I am eternally grateful for the direction and motivation she has given me, as well as her expert knowledge that has been invaluable in writing this book.

I have had the honour and privilege of training with some great Thai teachers and Masters of Traditional Thai Massage and my thanks go to Chongkol Setthakorn, Somphat, Mama Lek, Jack Chaiya, Nit Chaimonkol, Pichest Boonthume, the staff at the Old Medicine Hospital in Chiang Mai and TMC Chiang Mai, as well as the staff at Wat Pho. To these teachers I am very grateful along with the many Thai therapists who have shown me much along the way, especially Atchalee Siriwan (Angie) for her help and friendship.

My only Western teacher of Thai Massage was a German man by the name of Harald Brust, better known as Asokanada or Ashoka. Ashoka wrote the first book in the English language on Traditional Thai Massage called *The Art of Traditional Thai Massage*. I have borrowed his title for this book as a dedication to Ashoka, and also, as at the time of writing, this is the first book in English on Thai Foot Massage. Ashoka was an incredible man who elevated his own practice of Thai Massage to an art form, and was an inspiration to many. As neither a leader, nor a follower I found myself surprised at the strength of my desire to follow Ashoka. I had intended to study with him for a few days whilst he was in London, and a few days turned into a couple of weeks, but this was still not enough. When he left I immediately began to plan more training with him. It took over a year to organise, but I eventually managed to take my family halfway around the world to New Zealand where he lived. Ashoka had warned me that he was unwell, but when I arrived he was very weak and terminally ill with cancer. Ashoka had cut short a *vipasana* meditation retreat that he did every year for a month in the jungles of Thailand, as he found himself too ill to continue. He was later diagnosed with cancer and there was to be no cure or remission. After his death I was training with Pichest, an incredibly gifted Thai Massage therapist who still taught in the old oral tradition. Pichest was one of Ashoka's teachers and explained to me that there are many strong spirits in the jungle and that these spirits had caused Ashoka's illness. When a very weak Ashoka made the journey to Thailand to speak with Pichest and seek some treatment advice Pichest recommended a local Shamanic woman known as the "egg lady", who could remove these spirits from Ashoka. This was not the advice Ashoka was looking for and decided not to go. There was to be no second chance, or chance to reconsider, as both the egg lady and Ashoka passed away a few weeks later.

I recall this story to highlight the Traditions of Thai Medicine. Supernatural power is the first of 4 possible causes of illness according to Traditional Thai Medicine and the powerful spirits of the jungle are mentioned as one of these supernatural powers. Such concepts are hard to accept in the West, where scientific evidence is essential, but these traditions have continued for thousands of years in Thailand, and have survived the arrival of Western medicine. Traditional Thai Medicine has earned its right to exist and has proved its validity over the centuries. The current revival of Traditional Medicine has come about due to the need for a return to a holistic and proactive approach to the health of Thai people that Western medicine does not offer.

Thai Foot Massage is a part of Traditional Thai Medicine which has become immensely popular within the current revival of Thai Medicine. It contains enough elements of science to stand up under scientific scrutiny and also asks many questions that cannot be answered by science alone. This allows the experienced practitioner to perform the treatment as a healing art rather than a scientific therapy. I have taught this art to many and varied students, from the very physical approach of the sports masseur, to the esoteric approach of the modern day shaman. I can show a student how to practise techniques correctly and try to convey a feeling for the Thai culture and way of working. It takes time and practice to perfect Thai Foot Massage and begin to express this as art.

When I began teaching Thai Foot Massage I did not intend to write a book. Collating a manual had been difficult enough. However you can only be asked "Are any books available?" so many times, before you realise that one needs to be written. There were also courses on offer which taught versions of Thai Foot Massage that varied incredibly from anything I had received and been taught in Thailand. So as well as demand there also seemed to be the need to set the record straight on what exactly Thai Foot Massage is.

This book is intended to encourage anyone to learn Thai Foot Massage, to practise on friends and family and to help spread this healing art around the world. There are no prerequisites or entry requirements; all you need is someone to practise on. The only assessment you will undergo is the informal assessment of your volunteer.

Whether you are a practising therapist, or a complete beginner, I have tried to make this book an enjoyable read and a useful training tool with which to learn Thai Foot Massage. I have tried to give an insight into the Traditions of Thai Medicine to which Thai Foot Massage belongs. There is of course no substitute for learning from a teacher as a book can only show you so much. If you can, I suggest that you learn in Thailand, but if not at least learn from someone who has trained in Thailand and can give you an insight into the traditions of this powerful healing art. In this book I have brought together all of the techniques that I have learnt at many schools throughout Thailand, along with many techniques which I have picked up along the way from practising therapists.

My thanks go to my partner Paula, whose introduction to reflexology proved so alluring, and to our families on both sides of the world who have all helped in one way or another in the writing of this book. My thanks also go to my teachers and students who have enabled me to write this book.

Simon Piers Gall
November 2007, England

Part One

~

Theory

Introduction

What better way to health than to spend an hour of your time having your feet massaged? Traditional Western belief may hold that your hour would be better spent working out at the gym, or studying the dos, and don'ts of the latest diet craze. Not in Thailand, In Thailand you can have a "Foot Massage for Health"; it is not an act of pure self-indulgence to be accompanied by a feeling of guilt (although it does feel great), it is a complete and holistic treatment for your mind, body and spirit.

Eastern and Western philosophies have very different approaches to health. In the West we may take out medical insurance that we pay for whilst we are healthy, so that if we become unhealthy we will receive the best treatment money can buy in order to restore our health. Eastern philosophy will see you paying for treatment whilst you are healthy in order to remain healthy. Thai Foot Massage is arguably the most popular, but certainly the most visible part of this proactive approach to health in Thailand.

The name Thai Foot Massage is not completely accurate, as the massage is not only performed on the feet, but also on the lower leg. The conventional Western view of the massage would explain it in physiological terms as the manipulation of soft tissue and the mobilisation of joints; however in the East it is considered as much more. Apart from just feeling fabulous the massage also aims to stimulate the internal organs of the body via the reflex points of the feet. Reflex points are specific points on the foot that correspond to an internal organ. The massage also works along the energy (sen) lines of the feet and lower legs to balance and harmonise the flow of energy around the body. Sen lines are invisible channels that allow energy to flow throughout the body. This stimulation of the internal organs and the energy lines is intended to facilitate the body's normal functions and by doing so the body remains healthy.

This description immediately demands that you accept both the idea of reflex points on the feet and the existence of energy lines throughout the body. Neither of these theories forms a part of our biology lessons and there is no scientific proof of their existence according to conventional Western science. As you learn Thai Foot Massage it is not important whether you accept these theories or not, just to be aware of the theory is enough for now. When you can perform a massage without referring to this book you will have become at least competent in Thai Foot Massage and may have already received some remarkable feedback. When you can perform the massage using the expression of your intent you will have elevated it to an art form, and you will be able to gather your own anecdotal evidence of its benefits.

Thai Foot Massage is similar to reflexology as we know it in the West. In Thailand they would say "same same", which colloquially translated means similar, and not the same. This can be quite a frustrating concept when you are trying to be precise, but great if you are on holiday enjoying the relaxed or *sabai* attitude of Thailand.

The main differences between Thai Foot Massage and reflexology are that of the therapist's intention, and the emphasis of the massage. Reflexology, which means "the study of the reflex points" emphasises, as the name suggests, an examination of the reflex points, followed by a bespoke treatment intended to stimulate specific internal organs depending on the results of the reflexologist's examination. Christine Issel in her book *Reflexology: Art, Science and History* makes the following distinction: "Reflexology should not be confused with foot massage" and goes on to say "Reflexology makes use of very precise reflex points". Reflexology has progressed beyond massage and has become a tool, by which the advanced practitioner can assess the health of the internal organs of the body, by studying their corresponding reflex point on the foot, and even work to improve the health of these organs by working the reflex points of the foot.

Thai Foot Massage, on the other hand, emphasises the massage and is intended to generally stimulate the reflex points of the feet, in order to stimulate the internal organs generally and encourage the free flow of energy throughout the body by thoroughly massaging both the feet and the lower legs. Thai therapists rarely examine the reflex points during a massage, and perform their routine massage knowing that the techniques they employ

promote general health and well-being. The practice of keeping to
the routine does not necessarily detract from the treatment, and
can be quite refreshing. There is no appointment to make, or rush
to keep, no lengthy consultation or treatment plan. You merely
take a seat, put your feet up and *sabai* (relax)!

It is this general approach to the reflex points, the multitude of
massage techniques employed, and the working of the energy lines
that defines Thai Foot Massage and differentiates it from
Reflexology.

Thai Foot Massage is not a soft and soothing massage with
superficial techniques, but more a refreshing and revitalising
massage that is deeply relaxing. The therapist works to the beat of
their heart or to the rate of their breathing with a depth of pressure
to match.

This form of foot massage has been practised for thousands of
years and originated in India as part of the *ayurvedic* medical
system. The version that we see today in Thailand has evolved

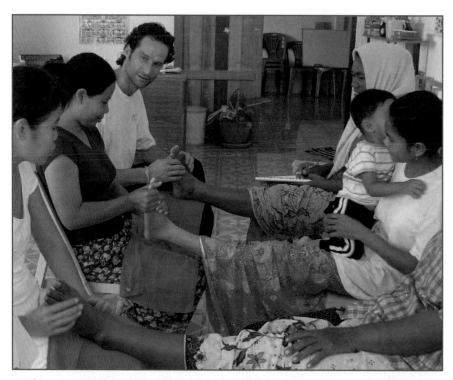

*Taking tea to China! Teaching Thai Foot Massage to some local villagers at
Ban Thalae Nok Community Centre on the Andaman Coast, as part of a
post Tsunami relief programme*

with both Indian and Chinese influence, along with other Far Eastern medical practices. This sharing of knowledge and techniques has been brought about by the spread of Buddhism and the many trade routes throughout Southeast Asia.

It is not, however, only the geographical location of Thailand between the two great nations of India and China that has allowed it to benefit from their medical systems. The nature of the people of Thailand, known as the "Land of Smiles" is very welcoming, hospitable and immediately endearing. This aspect of Thai culture has enabled them to benefit from the many welcome visitors. *Sawasdee*, meaning welcome, is a word that is unavoidable in Thailand and underlines their nature. This is ever present in the spas of Thailand, which are second to none. The relaxed yet attentive nature of Thai service flourishes in this environment. Pampering has a purpose in Thailand and that purpose is to promote good health.

Overview of Thai Traditional Medicine

In order to understand the phenomenon that Thai Foot Massage is today in Thailand it is necessary to understand its place within the holistic approach of Traditional Thai Medicine.

According to Traditional Thai Medicine the body is made up of four elements: earth, water, wind and fire. These elements are collectively known as *tard*. Of these elements each individual has a dominant element known as *tard chao ruan,* which is determined by the date and time of an individual's conception. This *tard chao ruan* will determine an individual's appearance and characteristics, as well as the vulnerable aspect of their health.

During an examination and diagnosis a practitioner will take a full consultation and perform a physical examination. They will determine your *tard chao ruan* to identify any imbalances in these elements and may also perform an astrological examination to determine the cause of illness.

Within Traditional Thai Medicine there are 4 possible causes of illness as highlighted by Vichai Chokevivat and Anchalee Chuthaputti in their paper *The Role of Traditional Medicine in Health Promotion*:

- **Supernatural powers,** e.g. ancestor's soul, powerful spirits of the forest, evil spirits, punishment from a heavenly spirit for those who misbehave.
- **Power of Nature,** e.g. imbalance of the four elements of the body (earth, water, wind, and fire).
- **Power of the universe,** e.g. influence of the sun, moon, and stars.
- *Kimijati,* or micro organisms and parasites of conventional Western medicine.

Treatment offered by Thai Traditional Medicine is split into 3 main areas:
- **Medicine,** including herbal remedies and traditional medicines.
- **Massage** *(nuad),* including Thai Foot Massage, Traditional Thai Massage, herbal compresses used alone or within a massage, and herbal steam baths.
- **Meditation** *(dhammanamai),* which encompasses Buddhist rites and meditation as well as living one's life on the "middle path" of Buddhism in order to avoid over- or under- indulgence. Eating a healthy diet, including appropriate herbs, and the practice of *ruesi dud ton* or *Thai Yogha* as a traditional form of meditative exercise.

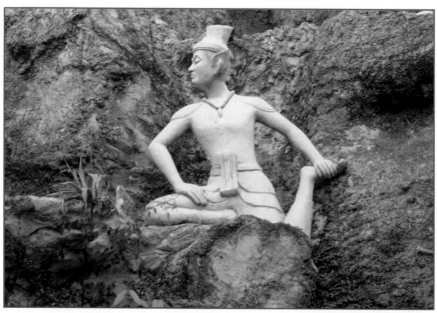

A reproduction of one of the original 80 Thai Yogha statues on display at Wat Pho

This holistic approach to the mind, body and spirit is proactive as Thai people are encouraged to maintain health by using herbs correctly in food, taking regular massage, and by following *dhammanamai* which is split into three categories:

- **Kayanamai** (healthy body) By practising *Thai Yogha,* and by having a good diet.
- **Jitanamai** (healthy mind) By practising meditation and studying the Buddhist teachings.
- **Chevitanamai** (healthy lifestyle) By following the "middle path" of Buddhism

It is the accessibility, as well as the benefits, of all aspects of Traditional Thai Medicine, and in particular Thai Foot Massage that has enabled it to become as popular as it is today. There is never a problem finding somewhere to have a Thai Foot Massage and so with this mass supply the question of "why" has been replaced with "why not"!

The History and Development of Thai Foot Massage

Ancient History

Thai Foot Massage is incredibly popular in Thailand today. On the tourist trails you are never far from somewhere offering you the chance to put your feet up and watch the world go by. Traditionally however, all forms of Traditional Thai Massage were seen as a spiritual practice, found in temples and hospitals, rather than the beach or the market place.

The tourist trade undoubtedly drives the huge number of people offering Thai Foot Massage, and, with a one hour massage costing the equivalent of a day's minimum wage, these shops remain focused on the tourist trade. Despite this, Thai Foot Massage still remains an integral part of the Thai Culture and way of life. It is commonly practised within the family and between friends for relaxation and health, as well as by traditional Thai doctors and healers.

Traditional Thai Massage credits an Indian Ayurvedic Doctor, known as Jivaka Kumarabhacca (c. 500 BCE), as the father or

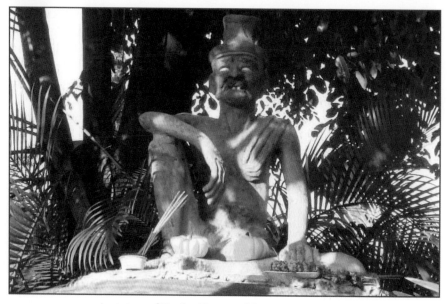

A statue of Jivaka Kumarabhacca at Wat Pho

founder of Traditional Thai Medicine. Prayers are made in his honour prior to a massage and his spirit is invited to work through the practitioner and guide their treatment. This prayer, known in Thailand as *Wai Kru* (honouring the teacher), is spoken in Pali and Sanskrit, two ancient Indian languages.

There are different versions regarding the birth of Jivaka Kumarabhacca, whose name translates as "to live" and "be raised by a Prince". All of the versions agree that Prince Abhaya adopted Jivaka. Prince Abhaya was the son of King Bimbisara of the Maghadan Empire (North Eastern India). As Jivaka grew he became interested in medicine and healing and spent seven years studying with a renowned Indian Doctor. By the time he had finished his study he had surpassed even his teacher and was sent out to practise with his teacher's blessing. His ability to heal was legendary and he became famous throughout India treating Kings and Princes. His most renowned, and favourite patient of all was the Buddha whom Jivaka attended three times a day. Jivaka even built a monastery in his garden and donated it to Buddha and his disciples.

After Buddha's death it was not until the reign of the Indian emperor Ashoka (c. 300 BCE) that Buddhism became established on a national level within India. Emperor Ashoka began to spread the teachings of Buddha internationally by sending Buddhist monks throughout Southeast Asia. These monks, who were often trained in Ayurvedic principles, not only spread the word of Buddhism, but also the now legendary stories of Jivaka Kumarabhacca and the Ayurvedic principles. The monks set up temples and hospitals wherever they settled and their skills became integrated with local medical practices. Thailand is thought to have had mainly shamanic style healing practices prior to the arrival of Buddhism.

The spread of Buddhism and the ancient trade routes of Southeast Asia show how Buddhism first spread from India towards China and then further East to Japan and Korea. It also shows how Buddhism spread back from Japan to Northern Thailand. This spread of Buddhism and the trade routes show the general direction of travel. The routes were not simply from A to B. Trade, along the Silk Road for example, did not involve taking goods from one end of the road to the other; goods were generally sold on along the way. Smaller routes branching from these main routes enabled local traders to join the route and became market places and stop off points. Although there is no evidence I would imagine that *Padabhyanga*, the ayurvedic name for foot massage, would have been a popular skill on such treks.

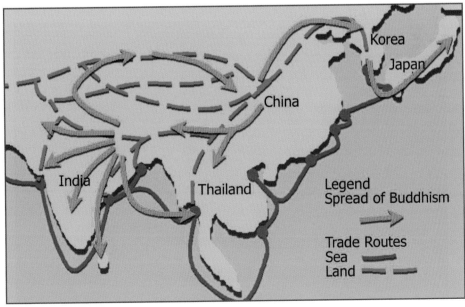

Map showing the spread of Buddhism and trade routes throughout SE Asia

The acknowledgement of Jivaka Kumarabhacca as the founder of Traditional Thai Medicine firmly roots the origin of this tradition in India however; other cultures and countries have also influenced the treatments that we see today in Thailand. For example the stick used to stimulate the reflex points in Thai Foot Massage originated in Taiwan as a tool for providing greater depth of pressure.

Christine Issel in her book *Reflexology: Art, Science and History*, describes two streams of reflexology converging in the West during the Middle Ages, one from the East (India) and one from the West (Egypt).

There is a famous image from Egypt that is credited as being the first image of Reflexology on the walls of Ankhamor's tomb dating back to 2330 BC, but as Christine Issel states "The art of reflexology was not only known in Egypt but it was also known 5,000 years ago in ancient India."

These two historic points of reference suggest that some form of foot massage may well have occurred simultaneously in two distant cultures, suggesting that maybe foot massage, by whatever name, is an archetypal form of massage with more than one origin. It is however the Eastern or Indian foot massage from which Thai Foot Massage originated.

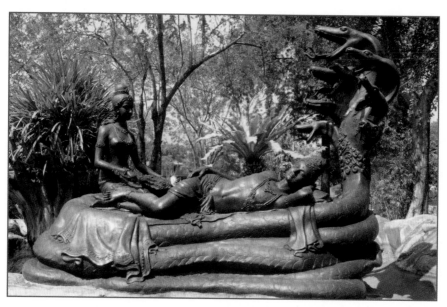

Thai image of Vishnu with Lakshmi at his feet

Within India the feet, or pada, have always been a focus of worship. Prior to Buddhism, Hinduism was the main religion of India, which predates Buddhism by at least 1,000 years. In Hindu tradition the contact of the feet with the earth enables the earths' energy to flow throughout the body and mind.

Hinduism celebrates many gods. The three most important are Brahma, the creator, Vishnu the preserver, and Shiva the destroyer. Vishnu the preserver is often depicted in Hindu art with Lakshmi massaging the feet of Vishnu. Lakshmi is Vishnu's Shakti, or female counterpart, and represents positive female energy.

An 18th Century drawing of the Feet of Vishnu places various symbols at specific points on the soles of the feet. There are some striking similarities in the placement of these symbols with some of the reflex points, although the meaning of the images is not clear. The points used in *Padabhyanga* are known as Marma points and although there are correlations between these Marma points and the reflex points of Thai Foot Massage the Marma points number far fewer than those used in Thai Foot Massage.

The footprints (padamudra) of gods have also been treated as objects of worship in Hinduism, and several temples have been built around these footprints throughout Southeast Asia. This tradition of worshipping the feet and footprints continued into Buddhism where worshipping the Buddha's footprints represents following the path of Buddha. These footprints are often depicted as having auspicious symbols on the soles of the feet, which represent the saintly life and teachings of Buddha.

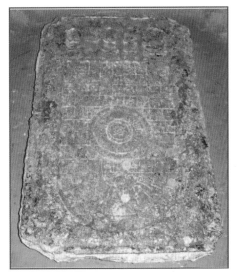

These images of Buddha's footprints are particularly popular in Thailand and are found wherever Buddhism spread, including China, Japan, and Korea.

China's influence on Thai Foot Massage is most evident in the maps of the reflex points that are used. These

An impression of Buddha's Footprint from Wat Phra Phuttabat, in Saraburi Province

maps are very similar and correspond almost entirely to some of the maps used in China.

Historical records of massage, and in particular foot massage, are few and far between, however there is enough evidence to surmise that foot massage was an integral part of the traditional medicine of India, China, and Thailand.

In China there are historical records written by Sima Qian referring to a well-known doctor during the second century BC called Yu Fu (meaning foot healing) who treated his patients purely by massaging their feet.

Also the book The Yellow Emperor's Classic of Internal Medicine, or Huangdi Nei Jing, which deals mainly with acupuncture (thought to have been written sometime between 475–221 BCE) identifies six important channels that travel to and from the foot, and identifies 66 points along these channels on the feet. The book does mention massage and, although foot massage is not mentioned specifically, the importance of the foot is emphasised by the concentration of points on the feet.

It may be that the massage techniques, or pressing and rubbing, as massage translates, remained as part of an oral tradition that were taught rather than studied as the written word. Such techniques don't lend themselves to wordy descriptions, and are much more easily taught by demonstration and practice.

Priority seems to have quite rightly been given to the points and the lines or channels of energy.

In Thailand, until very recently, all aspects of Traditional Thai Massage were taught in this oral tradition. Techniques were not recorded and records were not kept in written form. Students would traditionally learn as apprentices under the guidance of a Master. There was no syllabus to study, just the teachings of the master. A student would complete their apprenticeship when the master was satisfied that they were ready to practice their skills and continue the good reputation of the Master. This approach is potentially very good for an apprentice and this method has been responsible for adding to the variety and styles of Traditional Thai Massage. It has however meant that historical records were scarce.

Another reason for the lack of historical evidence in Thailand could be partly to do with the lack of original research. The reflex points for example, seem to have been, in the main, adopted from the Chinese. It is the many massage techniques that makes this treatment Thai, and historically massage techniques in general are not well documented.

Of the records still in existence regarding the broader tradition of Thai Medicine there is evidence of 102 hospitals, known as Arogaya sala, throughout the Khmer kingdom (Northeast Thailand) In 1238 CE during the Sukhothai period, suggesting that an indigenous form of healing was well established by this time.

During the Ayutthaya period (1350–1767) there were herbal drug dispensaries for the public as well as a royal drug dispensary in the royal palace, and later during the reign of King Narai the Great (1656–1688) the king's doctors wrote the first official book of Thai Herbal Medicine called *Tamra Phra Osod Phra Narai.*

Modern History

When the Burmese invaded Thailand in 1767, the old capital Ayutthya was ransacked and destroyed along with many sacred texts and records. Much of Thailand's cultural history was destroyed in this invasion. Following this invasion King Rama I, when he was crowned, moved the capital of Thailand to Bangkok or Krung Thep (City of Angels) as it is known in Thailand. Having proved himself as a great warrior during this invasion, he also proved to be a great and fair leader to his people. He began a process of restoration following the Burmese invasion, encouraging Thai literature and bringing together many remaining works of art and culture. In 1788 He began the building of Wat Phra Chetuphon on the grounds of two separate temples Wat Salak and Wat Phodharam, the latter was already

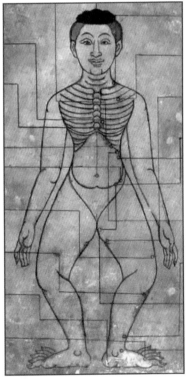

One of sixty stone inscriptions at Wat Pho, depicting the Sen lines of the body

known as a centre for education and learning of Traditional Thai Medicine. The King intended to compile the traditional knowledge of Thailand, and preserve it within the walls of the temple, so that it could be studied for the health of all the Thai people. There were no schools in Thailand at this time and temples were the main places of study. The temple is still commonly known as Wat Pho an abbreviation of Wat Phodharam, and is regarded by many as the home of Traditional Thai Massage. This restoration work took over seven years to complete.

Further restoration work lasting 16 years was made by King Rama III who had the walls of the temple covered with stone tablets inscribed with writings about various branches of Thai knowledge. These inscriptions were divided into eight groups. One of these groups deals entirely with herbal recipes and lists over 1,000 such recipes. Another section was dedicated to Thai Massage and Thai *Yogha* and originally showed 60 inscriptions of the energy (sen) lines of the body along with 80 statues showing Thai *Yogha* postures. Another part of this massive restoration work was the statue of the reclining Buddha. It is 46 metres long and 15 metres high. The most striking part of this statue, apart from the size, is the mother of pearl inlay depicting 108 auspicious symbols on the soles of the Buddha's feet in both Indian and Chinese styles.

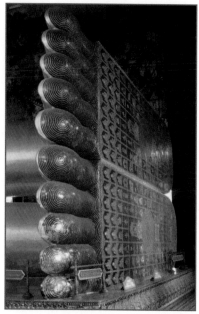

Image of Buddha's feet at Wat Pho

Thailand readily acknowledges that their Traditional Thai Medicine has been influenced by both the Indian and Chinese medical systems. Chokevivat and Chuthaputti in their article "The role of Thai Traditional Medicine in Health Promotion" describe Traditional Thai Medicine as involving medicine and massage, along with Buddhist rites and meditation, as well as rituals based on the belief in a supernatural power or the power of the universe. The article goes on to say that traditional knowledge was built up through the processes of "selection", "adoption", "adaptation" and "utilisation" of traditional medicine of some countries with which Thailand had contact in the past and mentions specifically India and China. These processes are still evident today with the most recent example being the Western influence on Traditional Thai Medicine. Since 1987 it has been possible to study and practice Applied Traditional Thai Medicine. An Applied Traditional Thai Medicine practitioner will use some western medical equipment to examine patients and decide whether modern or traditional medicine is most appropriate. Applied Traditional Thai Medicine practitioners can prescribe only traditional medicines or therapies to their patients.

Traditional Thai Medicine has evolved over the centuries and what we see today in Thailand are clear examples of both Chinese and Indian influence. However, Traditional Thai Medicine and Thai Massage stand as an entity on their own and cannot be understood by purely Chinese or Indian reference, or even by a combination of the two.

Eastern Philosophy Meets Western Science

Traditional Thai Medicine and Western medicine worked together briefly in Thailand but failed to become integrated, the traditional processes of selection, adoption, adaptation and utilisation were over ruled by Western medicine, and in the short term Western medicine completely replaced Traditional Thai Medicine

Missionaries and Doctors first introduced Western medicine to Thailand during the reign of King Rama III and, in 1888 Siriraj Hospital, the first western hospital and medical school was opened and taught Traditional Thai Medicine alongside Western medicine. The teaching of Traditional Thai Medicine was discontinued in 1916 when it was deemed to be incompatible with Western medicine as it relied too heavily on the doctors' opinion rather than scientific evidence. This was the start of a decline in Traditional Thai Medicine that was to last over 60 years.

The decline was compounded when in 1936 the "Control of the Practice of the Art of Healing Act" required practitioners of Traditional Thai Medicine to register and become licensed. Most practitioners did not register and so they became unlicensed and could no longer practice. Those that did become licensed had no place to practice, as western medicine had become the main form of treatment within hospitals. Traditional Thai Medicine was forced to retreat to poorer and rural communities where western medicine was unavailable.

It was not until 1978, when the World Health Organisation's Alma-Ata Declaration urged members to emphasise Primary Health Care to "protect and promote the health of all of the people of the world" that Traditional Thai Medicine began to recover. It was already evident that western medicine was failing the people of Thailand, the cost of expensive equipment and imported drugs left little for the prevention of disease and the promotion of health. Western medicine was also failing to cure several lifestyle related diseases such as diabetes, hypertension, cardiovascular diseases and various forms of cancer.

This World Health Organisation declaration sparked a resurgence of Traditional Thai Medicine that is still gaining momentum today. Medicinal plants are now at the forefront of Thai Medicine, and Traditional Thai Massage has benefited from the support of the government with national standards and curriculum being set by the Ministry of Public Health under the guidance of the Institute of Traditional Thai Medicine. In 1999 the Institute of Traditional Thai Medicine received a grant of 62 million baht from the Thai government to organise training courses in all aspects of Traditional Thai Massage and between 4,000 and 5,000 people were trained. This intensive training programme has led to the mass supply of Thai Foot Massage that is evident in Thailand today.

The Future of Thai Foot Massage

This huge supply of well-qualified Thai Foot Massage therapists has brought Thai Foot Massage out of the temples and hospitals and onto the promenades and street bazaars. Shops now offer treatments that would only be on offer in the best of western spas and the quality of these treatments has led to the demand for Thai therapists at some of the best spas around the world.

In the West complementary and alternative therapies generally take a more holistic approach than the clinical approach of conventional Western medicine, and already provide Primary Health Care with or without the official backing of their government. Many individual therapists and therapies have strived hard for recognition and acceptance from conventional Western medicine, and are having some success. Some techniques in isolation have been adopted in the West. Acupressure now appears as Neuromuscular techniques or trigger point work in massage, and Acupuncture has appeared as dry needling and been adopted by many Osteopaths and Physiotherapists. In these cases the whole concept of meridians and Traditional Chinese Medicine has not been adopted, but certain techniques have been borrowed. This convergence of ideas can only be a good thing for both conventional Western medicine and Complementary therapies.

The workplace has been fairly quick in adopting a proactive approach to the health of their workforce. Seated Acupressure Massage, for example, based on the Traditional Chinese Meridians has become very popular in the workplace of the Western world where we tend to hunch ourselves over computers and pay little attention to correct posture. Thai Foot Massage could also have a huge impact here. Workers who are not hunched over a computer tend to be on their feet all day, and Thai Foot Massage especially would be of great benefit in these circumstances.

Spas have also begun to look at their treatment menus. Spas and retreats used to be the realm of the rich and famous, but now the general population demand the same pleasures, but have a greater focus on value for money. Yes, the treatment must feel great, but it must also be good for their health. The latest addition to the spa world is the emerging market of the day spa and is reminiscent of the way Thai Massage is offered in Thailand. The day spa is beginning to head out from exclusive hotels and retreats to the High Street and shopping centres. The clientele do not expect miracle cures and are happy with anecdotal evidence rather than clinical studies that such treatments are good for you. People can spend a few hours in a tranquil setting and receive authentic and holistic treatments from around the world. As the popularity of Holistic therapies has grown, the general knowledge regarding the benefits of these treatments has also increased. The public not only want a treatment that will have a good effect, but it must also feel great. Thai Foot Massage is the original treatment to fit this bill, it feels undeniably good and it's good for you.

Perhaps in the not too distant future a Western Doctor will refer you for a course of complementary therapy. In the meantime however the market has begun to provide places where treatments are available to meet all your heart's desires, as well as all of your other organs!

How Thai Foot Massage Works

The Science and the Pseudo-science

There are many theories regarding the effect foot massage has on the body. The two theories that are most widely accepted have both a scientific and pseudo-scientific approach. The more scientific approach suggests that pressure applied to the 7,200 nerve ending in the feet stimulates an impulse along the peripheral nervous system. This impulse is then interpreted by the central nervous system, which in turn generates an impulse to create a motor response affecting the corresponding organ.

The Pseudo-scientific approach, which is of Eastern origin, suggests that the body has channels of energy flowing throughout the body, and that any blockages or stagnation of energy along these channels may result in illness or disease. Such blockages can be felt on the feet as lumps or crystals for example and, by massaging these points, blockages can be dissipated.

Thai Foot Massage follows the latter of these theories, which acknowledges the existence of energy channels within the body. As well as working the reflex points of the feet, Thai Foot Massage continues to work along the energy lines of the lower leg to encourage this flow of energy up and throughout the body.

This combination of massaging the reflex points of the feet and the energy lines of the legs adds a powerful dimension to Thai Foot Massage. Rather than hoping that the work that you have done on the foot flows through the body, you actively encourage the flow of energy by working the energy lines along the lower leg.

When you are enjoying a Thai Foot Massage it does actually seem a shame to stop at the knee. If Thai Foot Massage proves as addictive for you as it has for me, it may leave you feeling great but wanting more. Thailand has the answer again, in the form of Traditional Thai Massage.

My idea of a perfect day is to have a Thai Foot Massage followed by a full body Traditional Thai Massage with the use of Herbal compresses. The Thai Foot Massage stimulates your internal organs and begins to encourage the flow of energy throughout the body. The Traditional Thai Massage will then continue to open the energy lines from the tips of your toes to the top of your head (and out to each finger), by way of the therapist using various parts of their body to expertly stretch and compress you into various positions, so that this energy can flow freely. The use of the herbal compresses after a massage will have varying effects depending on the herbs used, however the generic compresses contain herbs that will detoxify the digestive system and relieve muscular tension. This would take up to about 3 or 4 hours of my perfect day, so I would have time left for some Thai food, where herbs are again used with expertise, and perhaps a dip in the Andaman sea! Of course ideally the rest of the day would involve some contemplation and meditation, as well as Thai Yogha, but I must remember that this is my perfect day and I am on holiday!

The Reflex Points of the feet

Being able to affect other parts of the body by massaging the feet is a very attractive idea, giving you the opportunity to be able to work on the shoulder, for example, without having to touch the shoulder, or stimulate the adrenal glands without open surgery. It is this access to the internal organs that is such a fascinating part of Thai Foot Massage.

The feet represent the entire body, with different areas corresponding to different areas of the body and specific points relating to specific organs.

Over centuries maps of the reflex points have been put forward and refined by different cultures and schools of thought. There are many more similarities than differences between these reflex maps, but differing schools of thought do occur between cultures and sometimes even within cultures.

These different opinions can become a major concern as to which map of these points is accurate and is often a topic for debate by reflexologists in the Western world. Here again Thai Foot Massage has its own set of maps which correlate and differ on some points.

The following maps show points that have been shown to me in Thailand. Again there are some differences and slight variations, however, with the general approach to these points within a Thai Foot Massage, it could be said that it is not so critical as to whether you are working on, for example the Thymus or Thyroid gland as it is all "good for you"! Of course for a more specific treatment this could be a major cause for concern.

Map Showing the Reflex Points of Thai Foot Massage

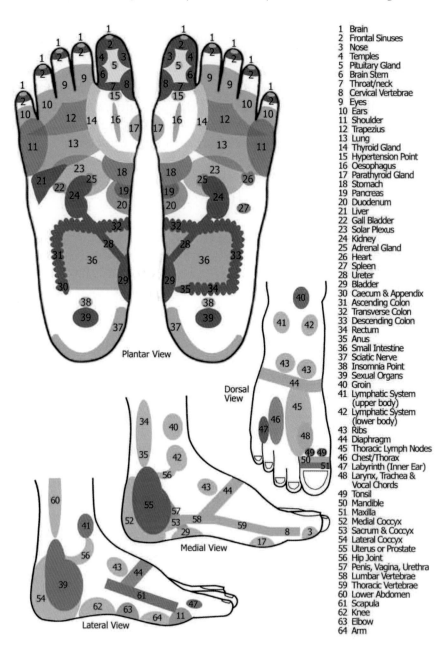

Plantar View

Dorsal View

Medial View

Lateral View

1 Brain
2 Frontal Sinuses
3 Nose
4 Temples
5 Pituitary Gland
6 Brain Stem
7 Throat/neck
8 Cervical Vertebrae
9 Eyes
10 Ears
11 Shoulder
12 Trapezius
13 Lung
14 Thyroid Gland
15 Hypertension Point
16 Oesophagus
17 Parathyroid Gland
18 Stomach
19 Pancreas
20 Duodenum
21 Liver
22 Gall Bladder
23 Solar Plexus
24 Kidney
25 Adrenal Gland
26 Heart
27 Spleen
28 Ureter
29 Bladder
30 Caecum & Appendix
31 Ascending Colon
32 Transverse Colon
33 Descending Colon
34 Rectum
35 Anus
36 Small Intestine
37 Sciatic Nerve
38 Insomnia Point
39 Sexual Organs
40 Groin
41 Lymphatic System (upper body)
42 Lymphatic System (lower body)
43 Ribs
44 Diaphragm
45 Thoracic Lymph Nodes
46 Chest/Thorax
47 Labyrinth (Inner Ear)
48 Larynx, Trachea & Vocal Chords
49 Tonsil
50 Mandible
51 Maxilla
52 Medial Coccyx
53 Sacrum & Coccyx
54 Lateral Coccyx
55 Uterus or Prostate
56 Hip Joint
57 Penis, Vagina, Urethra
58 Lumbar Vertebrae
59 Thoracic Vertebrae
60 Lower Abdomen
61 Scapula
62 Knee
63 Elbow
64 Arm

It is fairly clear, especially when you just glance at the maps of the feet, that wherever you massage the foot you will be massaging many reflex points and so affecting the corresponding body parts associated with these points.

Do not be concerned that you are stimulating organs that may not need stimulating, as Thai Foot Massage is like rain falling to the earth. The rain does not head for the dry soil in order to moisten it or to the flower to make it bloom, it just falls. The earth instinctively absorbs the rain or allows it to flow to where it is needed.

The Sen Lines or Energy Channels

The idea of invisible channels allowing energy to flow throughout the body is not unique to Thailand and occurs throughout Asia. In India the Ayurvedic principles of medicine call this energy prana, and refer to the channels through which this prana flows as nadis. In China the principles of Traditional Chinese Medicine call this energy Qi and refer to the channels as Meridians, and in Thailand the channels are known as Sen, and the energy is sometimes referred to as *lom*, or wind. These cultures all suggest there are 72000 energy channels throughout the body, although this has been suggested as a Buddhist pseudonym for countless rather than a precise figure.

Each culture has settled on a finite number of channels as being the main channels. Whilst there is again much common ground in the running of these channels there are also differences that are unique to each culture and also within each culture. The Thai system of Sen lines accepts 10 main Sen lines, known as "Sip Sen" (10 channels). My only Western teacher, Harald Brust, also known as Asokananda or Ashoka, did a great deal of research into sen lines and it is his charts of the energy lines that I use throughout my Traditional Thai Massage treatments, and in this book.

For the purposes of this book I have just shown the Sen lines of the lower legs as they are worked in a Thai Foot Massage.

Of the ten energy lines "Sip Sen" used in Traditional Thai Massage, we use six of these Sen lines during a Thai Foot Massage.

The Sen lines used are:

- Sen Sumana
- Sen Ittha and Sen Pingkala
- Sen Kalathari
- Sen Sahatsarangsi and Sen Thawari

Sen Sumana, is the equivalent, and namesake, of Sushumna Nadi of Ayurvedic Medicine and the Governing and Conceptual vessels of Traditional Chinese Medicine. Sen Sumana is considered the main energy line and runs up the centre of the body. This line runs up the back of the leg. Starting at the medial edge of the big toe, along the medial arch of the foot, around the heel, along the Achilles tendon, between the two heads of the Calf muscle (Gastrocnemius) to the centre of the back of the knee (popliteal area).

Good for: Abdominal and digestive disorders and back pain.

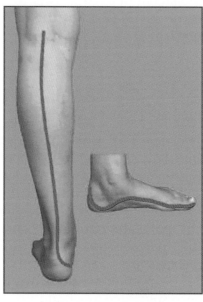

Diagram of Sen Sumana

Sen Ittha and **Sen Pingkala** follow the same route on opposite sides of the body. Sen Ittha is on the left side of the body, and Sen Pingkala is on the right side of the body. Sen Ittha relates to the moon and controls the left side of the body. This line is considered to have feminine qualities. Sen Pingkala relates to the sun and controls the right side of the body, and is considered to have masculine qualities. These two Sens again have a similar namesake in the nadis of Ayurvedic medicine, Ida nadi and Pingala nadi.

In Thai Foot Massage as well as Traditional Thai Massage you approach a man from his right side and a woman from her left side as these two lines should be worked according to their dominance. So with Thai Foot Massage you will generally start with the left foot for a woman and the right foot for a man.

These lines run from the lateral edge of the little toe, along the lateral edge of the foot and then up behind the lateral ankle and along behind the fibula to the bony protrusion at the top of the fibula.

Good for: Abdominal pain and back pain as well as all internal organs.

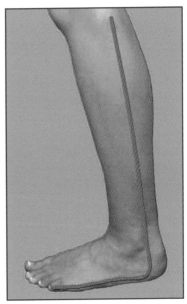

Diagram of Sen Ittha/Pingkala

Sen Kalathari, is known as the emotional or psychic Sen, and crosses the body from left to right at the abdomen and extends to our fingers and toes. This crossing of the Sen line allows the energy to flow from one side of the body to the other, helping to keep the two sides of the body in balance and harmony. This Sen runs through the centre of the medial head of the calf muscle reaching the foot midway between the medial ankle and the Achilles tendon. It then runs diagonally

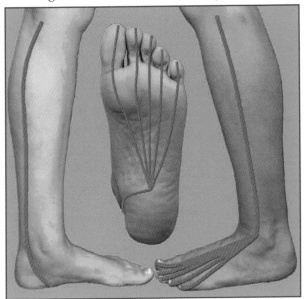

Diagram of Sen Kalathari

across the medial side of the heel and under the foot to the mid point along the top of the heel, where the heel joins the sole of the foot. From this point the line fans out into 5 branches that go directly to the tip of each toe. The line then continues over the top of the toes and along the dorsum of the foot, where the 5 branches begin to come back together as they travel up the dorsum of the foot and join again just in front of the lateral ankle. From here the line travels up onto the lateral side of the lower leg, just in front of the fibula bone and continues along next to the fibula to the top of the lower leg.

Good for: Keeping us "together" on an emotional level. Joint pains of the legs and feet, relieving physical tension brought on by emotional stress, and heart disease.

Sen Sahatsarangsi and **Sen Thawari,** like Sen Ittha and Sen Pingkala these Sen also follows the same route on different sides of the body. Sen Sahatsarangsi is on the left side of the body and Sen Thawari on the right side of the body.

These lines follow the lateral edge of the tibia, from the knee to the hollow where the leg joins the foot. From here the lines runs laterally across the dorsum of the foot to the lateral edge of the foot, and then under the foot, across the top of the heel like a stirrup to the medial arch of the foot. The line then comes just behind the medial ankle and follows the medial edge of the tibia to the top of the lower leg.

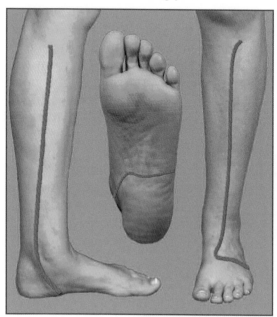

Good for: Knee pain and numbness of the legs.

Diagram of Sen Sahatsarangsi/Thawari

Part Two

~

Practice

Traditional Prayer for Healing and Guidance

Wai Kru

The following prayer or mantra is traditionally spoken prior to a massage as a way of paying respect to Doctor Jivaka Khumarabacca, and asking for his guidance during the massage. In my experience this prayer is not often spoken prior to a massage in the massage shops that exist today in Thailand, but would at least be spoken at the start of the working day.

It is written here phonetically so that you may use it.

Om Namo Jivaka Sirlasa Ahang Karuniko Sapasatanang
Osatha Tipi-Mantang Papaso Suriya-Jantang.
Khomalapato Pakha-Sesi Wantami Bandtito
Sumetaso A-rloka Sumnahomi

(3 times)

Piyo-Tewa Manussanang Piyo-Proma Namuttamo
Piyo Nakha Supananang Pininsiyang Namamihang
Namoputtaya Navon-Navien Nasatit-Nasatien
Ehi-Mama Navien-Nawae Napaitang-Vien Navien-Mahaku
Ehi-Mama Piyong-Mama Namoputtaya

(once)

Na-A Na-Wa Rokha Payati Vina-Santi

(3 times)

Original Sanskrit and Pali version:

We invite the spirit of our founder, The Father Doctor "Jivaka",
who taught us through his saintly life.
Please bring to us the knowledge of all nature,
that this prayer will show us the true medicine of the universe.

(3 times)

In the name of this mantra,
we respect your help and pray that through our bodies
you will bring wholeness and health to the body of our client.
The goddess of healing dwells in the heavens high,
while mankind stays in the world below.

In the name of the founder,
may the heavens be reflected in the earth below
so that this healing medicine may encircle the world.

(once)

We pray for the one whom we touch,
that he will be happy and that any illness will be released from him.

(3 times)

Translation by Chongkol Setthakorn

Setting the Scene

Things to Consider

This massage sequence will take about an hour and a half to complete once you know the treatment, and it will take longer whilst you are practicing. There is plenty of scope to shorten the treatment once you know the full routine properly, in Thailand it is generally offered for an hour. Whilst you are practicing you may prefer to perform just one section, and repeat this on both legs. It is better for both you and your partner if you perform a shorter treatment that is repeated on both legs, rather than trying to complete the whole massage but only managing one leg.

Preparing Your Room

Although Thai Foot Massage can be performed almost anywhere, and it often is in Thailand, it is best if you can work in private so that your client can relax totally. It is really up to you how you set up the room, but you should at least ensure that the room is warm and the lights are dimmed slightly.

Recliner chairs are generally used in Thailand, however, if you don't have a recliner chair don't worry, the massage can be performed on a couch, bed, or even the floor as long as you are both comfortable.

Make sure your partner understands that you are practicing and so the treatment may not flow completely to begin with. Both you and your partner need to have engineered enough time for the practice to be interruption free.

Things You Will Need

There is not really any specialist equipment needed for Thai Foot Massage. The Thai Foot Massage stick may be the only thing that is not to hand, but this can be replaced in the short term with the blunt end of a pencil or the first knuckle of your index finger. You will not need it until the second section, when we work on the reflex points, so that gives you time to practice the first section while you look for a suitable stick.

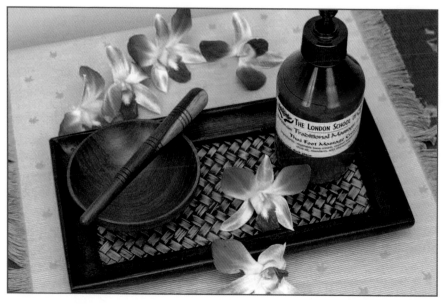

Thai Foot Massage stick with wooden bowl and tray

- *A pillow* – you may want to support your partners' feet and legs further with a pillow.
- *2 hand sized towels* – these will keep your pillow and chair clean and will also be needed later, at the end of the third section, to wrap up the feet and legs.
- *Cream and* oil – blend the cream and oil together in the ratio of about 3 parts cream to 2 parts oil. This can be done in a bowl just prior to the massage (your Thai Foot Massage stick makes a good stirrer), or can be pre-prepared. A mixture of cream and oil is used as oil is too slippery for this treatment and the skin absorbs cream too readily.

- *A large bowl of water and a flannel* – wash your partners' feet in the bowl, one at a time, before drying the feet and laying your partner back in the recliner. Apart from being a necessary hygiene precaution the washing of the feet at the start of a massage is very relaxing and is almost a ritual prior to the massage. I visited a small shop in Thailand where my feet were first soaked in a warm indoor waterfall and then scrubbed with salts, before being slowly walked along a short river to a recliner chair. Other places have merely brought out a damp cloth and wiped my feet clean. Aside from satisfying hygiene standards it is a great way to start a treatment and is worth performing well. Having said this I often use wet wipes when I am working away from home or teaching and they work just fine.

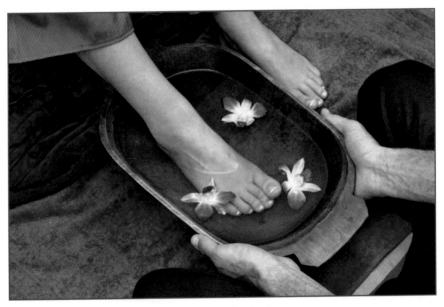

The feet are always washed prior to massage

The Consultation Process

A Thai foot Massage in Thailand will rarely involve a consultation, unless a Traditional Thai Medicine Practitioner is treating you. In the West, however a consultation should always be performed to at least rule out any total contraindications and make you aware of any cautions to the massage. With Thai Foot Massage it is possible to go through a checklist of contraindications and cautions to keep the consultation time to a minimum, but any questions that your partner raises should be answered and if you are in doubt as to whether to treat or not, you should always be prudent and not give them a massage.

Remember that this is not a diagnostic tool or a treatment for any condition.

Total Contraindications

If your partner is suffering from any of the following, you cannot massage them: *Infection; Disease; Fever; Under the influence of recreational drugs or alcohol; Diarrhoea; Vomiting; Pregnant (first trimester), or possibly pregnant.*

Medical Contraindications

If your partner is suffering from any of the following, your partner must first seek medical permission to have a massage: *Pregnant (second or third trimester); any cardio vascular conditions such as Thrombosis, Phlebitis, Hypertension, Hypotension, Heart Conditions; Haemophilia; Medical Oedema; Osteoporosis; Arthritis; Nervous or Psychotic conditions; Epilepsy; Recent operations; Diabetes; Asthma; Nervous system disorders; Trapped or pinched nerve; Inflamed nerve; Cancer; Kidney infections; Whiplash; Slipped or herniated disc; Acute rheumatoid arthritis.*

- Are you taking any prescribed medication?
- Are you being treated for any condition by another complementary therapist or Doctor?

Localised Contraindications

If your partner is suffering with any of the following, you must adjust your massage to avoid the affected areas: *Localised swelling or inflammation; Skin diseases; Varicose veins; Cuts or bruises; Recent scar tissue; Sunburn; Hormonal implants; Haematoma; Recent fractures; Cervical spondylitis; recent large meal.*

It is clearly possible from the above to make 3 lists of the contraindications in order to reduce the consultation time and merely check that there are no total or medical contraindications in order to proceed. There is also scope to increase the consultation to take in other factors such as emotional or lifestyle situations.

Finally the consultation should be signed and dated by your client, and any adjustments made to the treatment. These consultation forms should also be kept securely in order to maintain your partners' confidentiality.

After the Treatment

Getting Feedback

It is important for both your own practice and for your partners' comfort that you get feedback throughout the massage. Encourage them from the start to give you feedback, although if they fall asleep there is no need to wake them up for feedback! The Thai word for pain is "jeb" so make sure they let you know if they feel any "jeb". There should be no pain during the massage, even though some techniques can be fairly strong.

Feedback at some point after the massage is crucial to you developing a feel for the massage. This does not have to be straight after the massage, and can even be the next day or a few days later. Sometimes this is when you will get the most positive or negative feedback.

Also try to evaluate your own massage and consider which techniques worked well, which ones you liked and also which ones you disliked. If there are techniques that you disliked, ask yourself why and check as to whether you were performing the technique correctly.

Aftercare Advice

It is important that your partner has the time and space to relax after a treatment, they should not be rushing off to make up for the time they have been resting. In Thailand they will often give you a herbal tea and let you remain seated and relax for a while.

Even if the therapist has another customer there is always somewhere for you to sit.

This herbal tea is great, but if you do not have herbal tea at least get your partner a glass of water, and advise them to avoid alcohol or caffeine.

The Rhythm and Technique of Thai Foot Massage

The rhythm and the way the techniques are performed are perhaps the most important part of a good Thai Foot Massage. The two most important things to remember are to use your body, and work to the beat of your heart, and in time with your breathing.

Technique

When you begin to use the weight of your body to perform a massage you will immediately notice how effortless it is. Even when you are using your hands you will find that you no longer need to squeeze with the muscles of the hands and forearm. Instead you place your thumbs, or whichever part of your body the technique requires, onto the foot and then rock forward and lean onto your thumbs so as to add the pressure of your body weight rather than muscular force. This is an incredibly efficient way to work and saves a lot of energy. In Thailand a therapist may be working all day and be seeing clients one after the other. Without using your body this would be a very difficult task. When the technique is performed correctly your partner should feel a gradual increase in pressure as you lean or rock forwards and a gradual decrease in pressure as you rock backwards.

Use the pads of your thumbs rather than the tip of your thumb, and place your fingers on the foot to offer some support to the thumb.

Rhythm

If you get the rhythm wrong you will become fatigued very quickly. Thai therapists work to the natural beat of their hearts and keep their breathing in time with their heart. By keeping to this rhythm you will not overexert yourself or become tired. As you perform the rocking technique described above try to rock forwards on your heart beat and then rock backwards on the next heart beat.

And finally...

It is essential that you take notes as you practice. Whilst working through this book, remember that it is yours, put your name on it and make notes wherever you want to, sometimes a few arrows of your own design will make more sense to you than mine!

Each technique is named and numbered and should go some way towards describing the technique. The pictures will help and then below the 'How to...' section describes exactly how to perform the technique.

The reflex points and Sen lines worked in each technique are shown below the title, and at the end of each technique there is a boxed section describing the intention.

Whilst you are learning the techniques repeat each technique as many times as it takes for the technique to become familiar and feel natural.

I am often asked how many times should I repeat each technique, and admittedly I never count, but a general guide is approximately 10 times for the shorter techniques, and 3–5 times for the longer techniques. I have indicated, as a guide, how many times to repeat each move. Where there is no indication of repetitions, perform the technique once. Variations on this guide can also be used to lengthen or shorten the massage.

The Opening Sequence

This section begins to warm the foot firstly without any cream so that your intention is to work deeply and into the bones of the foot and then, once the cream is applied, you begin to warm the skin. There is a lot of work in this opening sequence to relax your partner both physically and emotionally.

This section works both the sen lines and the reflex points and is intended to warm up both in preparation for the more specific work later.

It is an incredibly thorough warm up and is a great way to start. I would suggest that, initially you complete this section on one foot and then repeat it on the other foot, before you start the other sections. Once you have gained experience you will complete the first three sections on one leg before beginning on the other leg.

Take time to relax and focus on your client before you start and you may perform the Wai Kru (page 32) if you wish.

When you feel relaxed and ready to begin, start on the left foot for a woman, or the right foot for a man, in order to focus on the dominant energies of Sen Ittha/Pingkala first. This book shows me working on the left side.

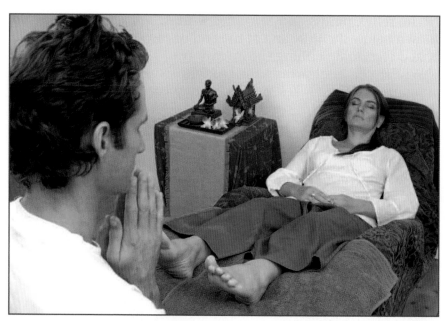

Time to focus and relax before you begin

Massaging without Cream

1 ~ Thumb Press Sen Kalathari on the Outside of the Leg

Sen Line – Kalathari.
Reflex Points – lymphatic system (upper body) and hip joint.

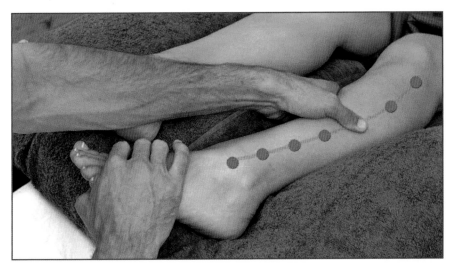

How to...

- Using your right hand, turn the left foot gently toward the midline so that the outside of the lower leg is more visible.

- Hold the foot with your right hand and with your left hand thumb press every couple of inches up, and then back down Sen Kalathari on the outside of the lower leg, this sen line runs from in front of the ankle and along above the fibula.

Intention

- The working of Sen Kalathari is intended to calm your client on an emotional level, and physically calm the heart and lungs and relax the limbs.

- Working the Reflex points of the upper lymphatic system is intended to encourage the return of lymph to circulation and encourage the lymphatic system to fight infection.

- Working the hip joint is intended to ease tension in this area and relax your client into the chair.

Remember...

Set the tempo of the massage and gently rock forward using your body weight to create the pressure of the thumb press, rather than squeezing with the hand.

2 ~ Thumb Press Sen Kalathari on the Dorsum of the Foot

Sen Line – Kalathari and Ittha/Pingkala.
Reflex Points – Lymph nodes (chest), chest, labyrinth (inner ear), ribs, diaphragm, larynx, trachea and vocal cords, and hip joint. On Sen Ittha/Pingkala – Shoulder, knee, elbow and arm.

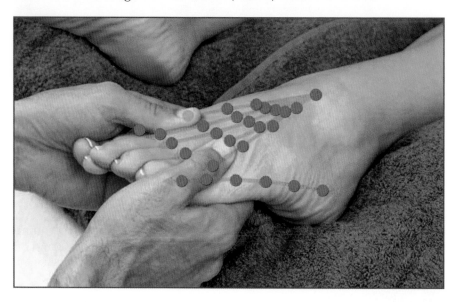

How to...

• Hold the foot in both hands with your thumbs on the top of the foot (dorsum) and your fingers on the sole of the foot.

• Starting in the channels between the first knuckle of the toes. Thumb press along 2 of the channels between the metatarsals of the foot to the depression or hollow in front of the ankle, and then back to between the first knuckle of the toes. Thumb press 2 channels at a time.

• Now repeat for the next 2 channels.

The Opening Sequence

- The fifth channel runs from the lateral edge of the little toe to the hollow in front of the ankle. Thumb press this channel from the toe up to the hollow and then back to the toe.

- Then thumb press along the lateral edge of the foot towards the heel along Sen Ittha.

Intention

- The working of Sen Kalathari is intended to calm your client on an emotional level, and physically calm the heart, lungs and chest.

- Working these reflex points will relieve tension in the chest area and relax the breathing as well as relaxing the limbs.

3 ~ Thumb Press Sen Ittha/Pingkala

Sen Line – Ittha (left leg); Pingkala (right leg).
Reflex Points – Sexual organs, lower abdomen.

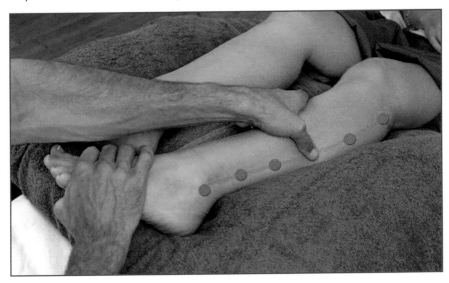

How to...

- Continue to hold the foot turned towards the midline, as before, and thumb press with your left hand up and then back down Sen Ittha, which runs from behind the ankle and along behind the fibula.

Intention

- Working Sen Ittha/Pingkala will relax all the internal organs and specifically relieve the lower back and abdominal area. This Sen also relieves tension of the head, neck and shoulders.

- Working the reflex points of the genitals and abdomen will help to stimulate and relieve any tension in this area.

4 ~ Thumb Press Sen Kalathari on the Inside of the Leg

Sen Line – Kalathari.

Reflex Points – Uterus or prostate gland, anus and rectum.

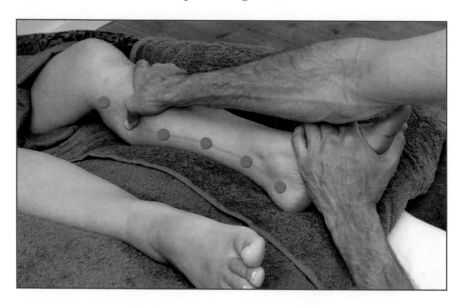

How to...

- Now change hands so you are holding the foot in your left hand, and turn the foot gently outwards so that the inside of the leg is more visible.

- Using your right hand thumb press up and then down Sen Kalathari. This line starts between the medial ankle and the Achilles tendon and runs up through the belly of the medial head of the calf muscle.

Intention

- The working of Sen Kalathari is intended to calm your client on an emotionally level, and physically calm the heart and lungs and relax the limbs.

- Working the reflex points of the uterus or prostate gland and the anus and rectum is intended to stimulate these organs and help your client let go of emotional tension.

5 ~ Thumb Press the Medial Arch of the Foot

Sen Line – Sumana.

Reflex Points – Nose, parathyroid, cervical vertebrae, thoracic vertebrae, lumbar vertebrae, sacrum and coccyx, uterus or prostate.

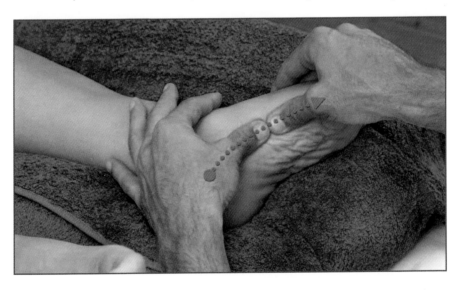

How to...

- Working with both thumbs tip to tip, thumb press with both thumbs from the heel, along the medial arch of the foot up to the big toe and along the medial edge of the big toe.

- Then thumb press back to the heel.

Intention

- Working Sen Sumana is intended to release tension in the chest, assist breathing, and also relieve tension in the back.

- Working the reflex points of the entire spine continues to help your partner relax into the chair and by stimulating the parathyroid gland assists the regulation of calcium in the blood for optimal bone formation and nerve function.

6 ~ Finger Circle Both Sides of the Heel

Sen Line – Ittha/Pingkala laterally (outside of foot) and Sumana medially (inside of foot).

Reflex Points – Coccyx, sexual organs, uterus or prostate.

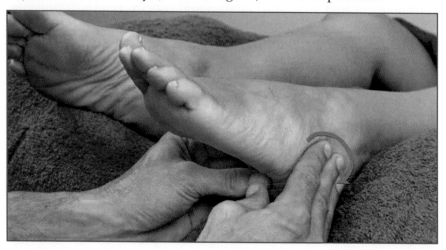

How to…

- Using the pads of the fingers of both hands, press and circle the skin to the inside and outside of the heel.

- Repeat 10 times.

Intention

Working Sen Ittha/Pingkala along with Sumana along with the reflex points of the coccyx will primarily assist in relaxing the back and specifically the lower back.

The Opening Sequence

7 ~ Palm Squeeze Both Sides of the Foot

Sen Line – Ittha/Pingkala (laterally) and Sumana (medially).
Reflex Points – Parathyroid, cervical vertebrae, thoracic vertebrae, lumbar vertebrae, sacrum and coccyx (medially); shoulder, arm, elbow, and knee (laterally).

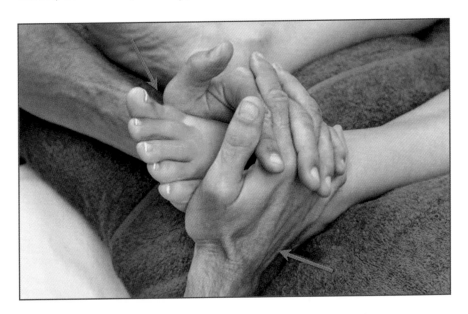

How to...

- Interlock your fingers and place your hands on top of the foot so that the heels of your hands cover the medial and lateral edge of the foot.

- Lift your elbows whilst keeping the heels of your hands against the edges of the foot, so that your wrists flex.

- Keep the wrists flexed and lower your elbows so that the heels of the hands squeeze the medial and lateral edge of the foot.

- Rock forwards in your chair as you squeeze the foot and rock backwards as you release.

- Repeat 5 times working up and down covering both the inside and outside edge of the foot.

NB: Squeeze should be created by rocking and lowering the elbows, not by muscular force.

Intention

Working Sen Ittha/Pingkala along with Sumana and the reflex points of the spine and limbs is primarily concerned with resting the spine and the limbs and encouraging the optimal function of the parathyroid gland.

8 ~ Rub the Ankle

Sen Line – Sumana, Kalathari, Ittha/Pingkala, Sahatsarangsi/ Thawari.

Reflex Points – Hip joint, uterus or prostate, sexual organs.

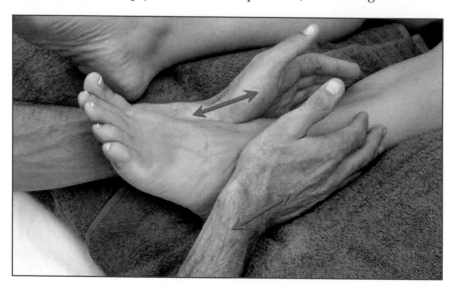

How to...

- Place one hand over the inside of the ankle and the other over the outside of the ankle so that the ankle is in the palm of the hands.
- The heel of your hand should be just cupping the ankle below the bone.
- Rub one hand forward as you rub the other back and repeat 10 times.
- The foot should wave or wiggle.

NB: Try not to slide your hands on the skin – hold the foot so that you are working in towards the joint.

Intention

This technique deeply relaxes the leg and the hip joint. All of the energy lines pass through the ankle joint and by releasing tension in this joint you allow the energy to flow more freely throughout the body.

9 ~ Foot Rub

Sen Line – Ittha/Pingkala (laterally) and Sumana (medially).
Reflex Points – Parathyroid, cervical vertebrae, thoracic vertebrae, lumbar vertebrae, sacrum and coccyx (medially); shoulder, arm, elbow and knee (laterally).

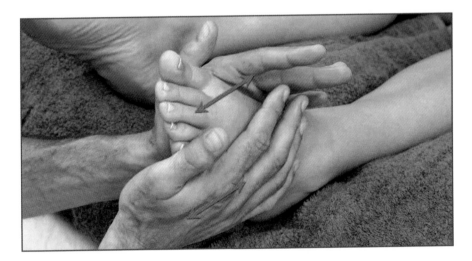

How to...

- Using both hands, hold the foot between your hands so that the inside and outside edges of the foot are near the base of your fingers.
- Rub forwards and backwards as you did for the ankle rub (number 8) – again not sliding on the skin, but working deeper into foot, loosening the bones and joints.
- Repeat 10 times.

> **Intention**
>
> Similar to the Palm Squeeze (number 7), but working with the fingers offers a more specific contact with each vertebra and limb.

10 ~ Thumb Press the Centre Line on the Sole of the Foot

Sen Line – Kalathari and Sahatsarangsi/Thawari.
Reflex Points – Sexual organs, insomnia point, sigmoid colon (left foot), small intestines, transverse colon, kidney, solar plexus, lung.

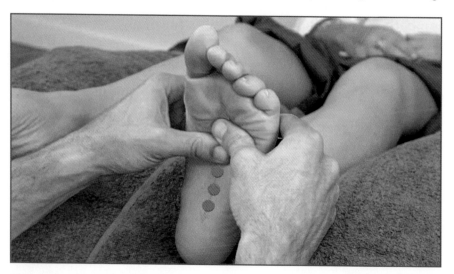

How to...

- Place both thumbs, one above the other at the centre of the heel on the sole of the foot.

- Gently rest your fingers on the dorsum of the foot.

- Rock forwards as you thumb press into the heel with both thumbs and rock backwards as you release.

- Move the thumbs slightly higher and continue up to the ball of the centre toe.

- Repeat coming back down the centre line of the foot.

- Repeat thumb pressing up and down 5 times.

Intention

Sahatsarangsi/Thawari is touched here to assist the function of the knee joint. The main work is on Sen Kalathari and the reflex points it covers. The intention here is to begin to encourage the energy to flow from the feet up through the body.

Massaging with Cream

11 ~ Apply Cream to Top and Bottom of Foot

Sen Line – Sumana, Kalathari, Ittha/Pingkala, Sahatsarangsi/ Thawari.
Reflex Points – All superficially.

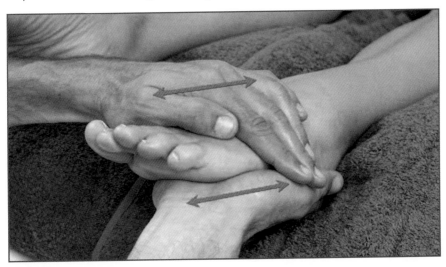

How to...

- Apply a scoop of cream to your hands, and warm the cream in your hands by silently circling the palms together.

- Clasp your hands together as if you had just clapped, or were about to rub your palms together in glee!

- Then open your hands as you slide your fingers and then your palms down the foot, with one hand on top of the foot and the other on the sole of the foot.

- Stroke all the way down to the ankle and then slide back up with some pressure and release.

- Now turn the hands as if to clap with the other hand on top and repeat.

- Repeat and alternate 10 times.

Intention

To warm the foot, reflex points, and sen lines, in preparation for the next section.

12 ~ Apply Cream to Achilles

Sen Line – Kalathari, Ittha/Pingkala, Sahatsarangsi/Thawari, Sumana.

Reflex Points – Uterus or prostate, rectum, coccyx, sexual organs, lower abdomen.

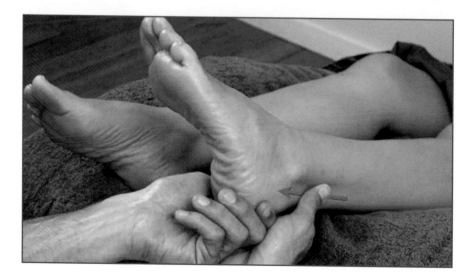

How to...

- Apply some more cream to your hands and then apply this cream to the Achilles tendon and heel with alternate hands.

Intention

To warm the back of the heel in preparation for later techniques and to relax the lower abdomen and further relax the ankle joint.

13 ~ Thumb Slide up Sen Kalathari on the Sole of the Foot and Flick off the Toes

Sen Line – Kalathari.

Reflex Points – Sexual organs, insomnia point, sigmoid colon (left foot), small intestines, transverse colon, kidney, solar plexus, adrenal gland, lung, trapezius, ear, eye, thyroid, throat/neck, head, pituitary gland, frontal sinuses, heart (left foot) liver and gall bladder (right foot), brain, oesophagus, hypertension point, shoulder.

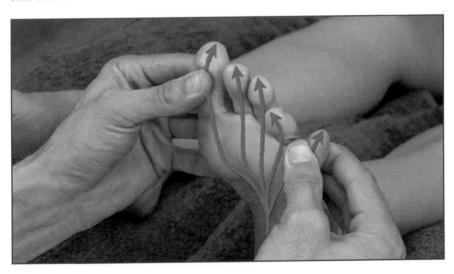

How to...

- Place both thumbs at the centre of the heel, one slightly higher than the other, and rest your fingers on the top of the foot.

- As you rock forward thumb press on the centre of the heel and then as you rock backward slide both thumbs up the centre of the foot and off the centre toe.

- Start again from the centre of the heel and slide both thumbs up the sole of the foot, but this time the thumbs spread at the beginning of the balls of the toes and flick off the 2nd and 4th toes.
- Repeat again and flick off the little and big toes.
- Now work your way back in by sliding up and off the 2nd and 4th toes and then the centre toe.
- Repeat 10 times.

Intention

To stimulate the flow of energy throughout the foot and up throughout the body.

14 ~ Thumb Slide down the Centre Line and off at either Side of the Heel

Sen Line – Kalathari, Sahatsarangsi/Thawari.
Reflex Points – Lung, adrenal glands, solar plexus, kidneys, transverse colon, small intestines, descending colon (left foot) ascending colon (right foot), rectum and anus (left foot), urinary tract and bladder.

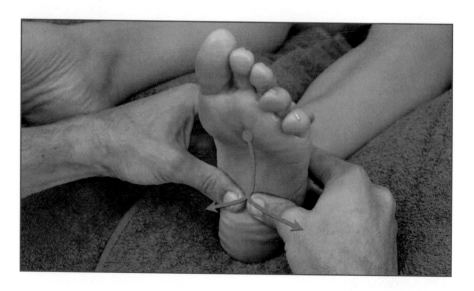

How to...

- Place your thumbs just below the ball of the centre toe, one slightly higher than the other, with your fingers resting on top of the foot.

- As you lean forward press with your thumbs and slide both thumbs down the centre line of the foot.

- At the top of the heel slide the thumbs out to each side so that they flick off to either side of the heel.

- Repeat 10 times.

Intention

To generally stimulate the flow of energy throughout the body and encourage elimination of stagnant energy by stimulating the bladder, the rectum and anus (left foot) and the ascending colon (right foot).

15 ~ Thumbs Criss Cross the Sole of Foot from the Centre Line

Sen Line – Kalathari, Sahatsarangsi/Thawari.

Reflex Points – Sexual organs, insomnia point, large intestine, small intestine, bladder, kidney, ureter, adrenal gland, pancreas, stomach, duodenum, solar plexus, shoulder, lung, trapezius, thyroid, ear, heart (left), spleen (left), liver (right), gall bladder (right).

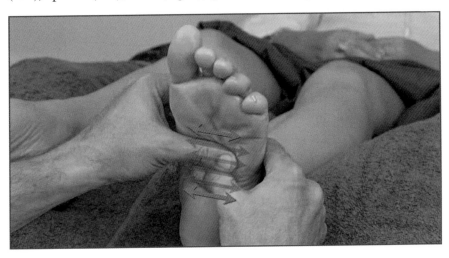

How to...

- Starting at the centre of the heel with one thumb slightly higher than the other.

- Press in as you rock forward and slide the thumbs out to each side.

- Return your thumbs to the centre line a little higher than before, with the other thumb higher this time and repeat.

- Continue to the balls of the toes and then work back down to the heel

- Repeat 10 times.

> **Intention**
>
> To stimulate many organs and encourage energy flow throughout the internal organs.

16 ~ Knuckle Slide the Medial Arch of the Foot

Sen Line – Sumana.

Reflex Points – Cervical, thoracic, lumbar and sacral vertebrae, and coccyx, penis or vagina, uterus or prostate, bladder, parathyroid gland.

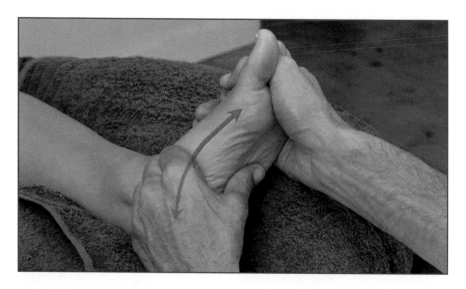

The Opening Sequence

How to...

- Hold the foot in your right hand with your thumb between the big toe and second toe.

- Turn the foot laterally so that you can see the medial arch of the foot.

- With your left hand slide the distal knuckles down the medial arch of the foot, from the big toe to the heel.

- Use the thumb of your left hand as a pivot point or guide as you slide your knuckles down the medial arch.

- Repeat 10 times.

Intention

To further relax the spine and encourage the energy of the base chakra to rise through the body.

17 ~ Knuckle Slide the Medial Side of the Heel

Sen Line – Sumana.

Reflex Points – Bladder, urethra and penis or vagina, sacrum and coccyx, uterus or prostate.

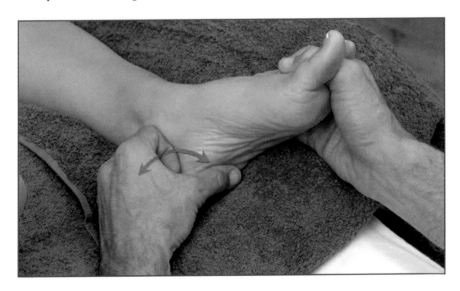

How to...

- Place the thumb of your left hand on the bottom of the heel of the foot and your knuckles on the medial side of the foot midway between the heel and ankle.

- Using your thumb as a pivot point, slide your knuckles across this part of the heel, working away from you.

- Repeat 10 times.

Intention

To further awaken and encourage the flow of energy from the base chakra.

18 ~ Knuckle Behind the Medial Ankle and Tibia

Sen Line – Sahatsarangsi/Thawari.

Reflex Points – Uterus or prostate gland, rectum and anus.

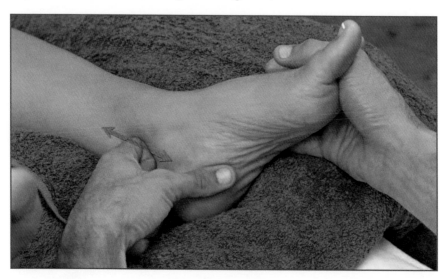

How to...

- Using the second knuckle of the first finger. Knuckle behind the medial side of the ankle and next to and behind the tibia.

- Place your thumb on the heel and use it as a pivot.

- Rock forward as you slide the knuckle up behind the ankle and the tibia, and then rock back as you slide the knuckle down with some pressure.
- Repeat 10 times.

NB: The uterus or prostate area can be quite sensitive so be aware of your clients' comfort and be sensitive.

Intention

More awakening of energy at the base of the spine.

19 ~ Chinese Burn to the Medial Arch of the Foot

Sen Line – Sumana.
Reflex Points – Cervical, thoracic, lumbar and sacral vertebrae and coccyx, penis or vagina, bladder and parathyroid.

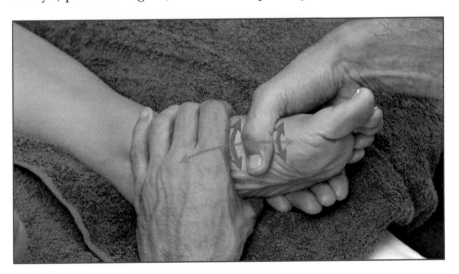

How to...

- Hold the medial arch of the foot with both hands, side by side. With your fingers on the dorsum of the foot and the thumbs on the sole of the foot.
- Grip the foot with both hands and then wring the foot working up and down the medial arch of the foot.

- As one hand moves forward the other hand should be moving backwards as if wringing a wet cloth.

- Repeat 3 times.

> **Intention**
>
> This technique allows for individual attention to each vertebrae and encourages the energy to rise from the base of the spine up through the body.

20 ~ Knuckle Slide the Lateral Edge of the Foot

Sen Line – Ittha/Pingkala.
Reflex Points – Shoulder, arm, elbow and knee.

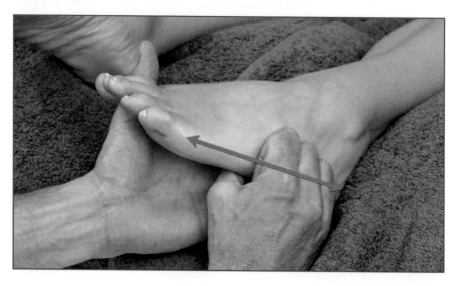

How to...

- Hold the foot in your left hand with your thumb between the big toe and second toe.

- Turn the foot medially so that you can see the lateral edge of the foot.

- With your right hand slide the distal knuckles down the lateral edge of the foot from the little toe to the heel.

- Use the thumb of your right hand as a pivot point or guide as you slide your knuckles down the lateral edge.

- Repeat 10 times.

Intention

To encourage your client to let go of any tension in their arms and legs by relaxing the limbs.

21 ~ Knuckle Slide the Lateral Side of the Heel

Sen Line – Ittha/Pingkala.
Reflex Points – Knee, sexual organs.

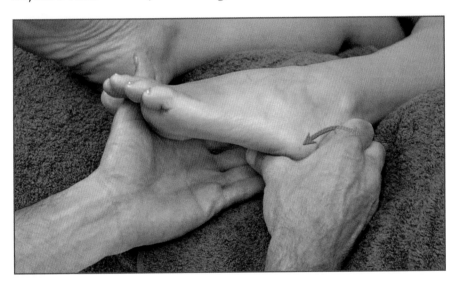

How to...

- Place the thumb of your right hand on the bottom of the heel of the foot, and your knuckles on the lateral side of the foot midway between the heel and ankle.

- Using your thumb as a pivot point, slide your knuckles across this part of the heel, working away from you.

- Repeat 10 times.

Intention

To awaken the energy at the base of the spine.

22 ~ Knuckle Behind the Lateral Ankle and Fibula

Sen Line – Ittha/Pingkala.
Reflex Points – Sexual organs, lower abdomen.

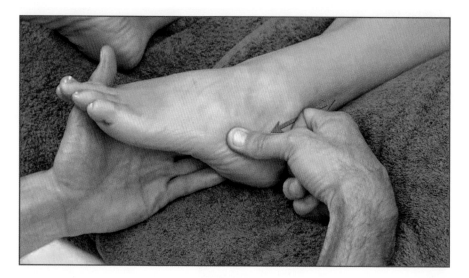

How to…

- Using the second knuckle of the first finger, knuckle behind the lateral side of the ankle and next to and behind the fibula.

- Place your thumb on the heel and use it as a pivot.

- Rock forward as you slide the knuckle up behind the ankle and the fibula and then, rock back as you slide the knuckle down with some pressure.

- Repeat 10 times.

Intention

To release emotional tension often held in the lower abdomen, and by doing so relaxing the lower back.

23 ~ Chinese Burn to the Lateral Edge of the Foot

Sen Line – Ittha/Pingkala.

Reflex Points – Shoulder, arm, elbow, knee.

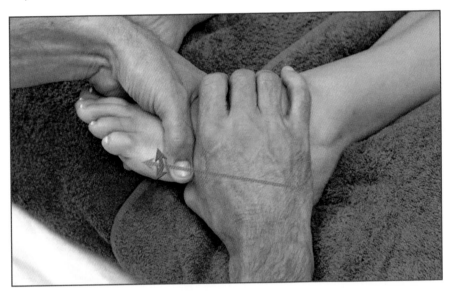

How to...

- Hold the lateral arch of the foot with both hands, side by side. With your fingers on the dorsum of the foot and the thumbs on the sole of the foot.

- Grip the foot with both hands and then wring the foot working up and down the lateral arch of the foot.

- As one hand moves forward the other hand should be moving backwards as if wringing a wet cloth.

- Repeat 3 times.

Intention

Encourage the flow of energy and deeply relax the limbs.

24 ~ Knuckle Slide Both Sides of the Ankle

Sen Line – Sumana, Kalathari, Ittha/Pingkala, Sahatsarangsi/ Thawari.
Reflex Points – Sexual organs, and hip joint (laterally). Hip joint, and uterus or prostate (medially).

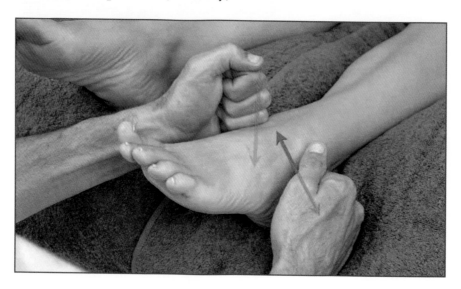

How to…

- Let go of the foot and make fists with both hands.
- Place one fist on the inside of the ankle and one fist on the outside of the ankle.
- Using the first knuckle of all the fingers, rub the hands up and down the inside and outside of the ankle.
- As one hand rubs up the other hand rubs down.
- Repeat 10 times.

Intention

Awaken further and encourage the flow of energy up through the trunk of the body.

25 ~ Knuckle Halfway around Both Sides of the Ankle

Sen Line – Shatsarangsi/Thawari, Ittha/Pingkala.
Reflex Points – Rectum and anus, uterus or prostate, hip joint, lymphatic system (lower body), (medially). Sexual organs, lower abdomen, hip joint, lymphatic system (upper body) (laterally).

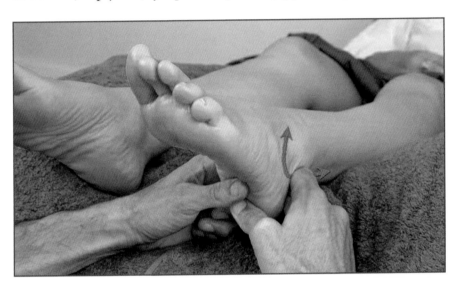

How to...

- Using the second knuckle of the index finger of both hands, knuckle half way around the inside and outside of the ankle at the same time.

- Place your thumbs on the heel of the foot for support.

- Starting behind the inside and outside of the ankle, slide the first knuckle of the index fingers up along, and behind the tibia and fibula as you rock forward.

- Slide the knuckles back down with some pressure as you rock backwards.

- Slide the knuckles below and around the inside and outside of the ankle so that they meet at the hollow at the top of the foot, as you rock forward.

- Slide the knuckles back down with some pressure as you rock backwards.

- Repeat 10 times.

The Opening Sequence

Intention

To awaken and further encourage the flow of energy around the ankle joint as well as stimulating the reflex points.

26 ~ Knuckle Slide the Achilles

Sen Line – Sumana.
Reflex Points – Rectum and anus, lower abdomen.

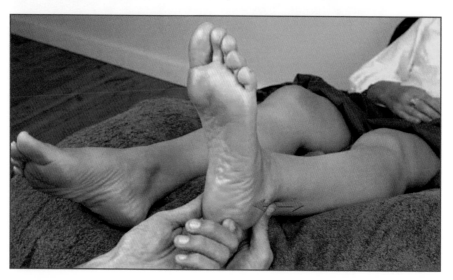

How to...

- Support the foot in your left hand so that it is held slightly above the cushion.

- Using the pad of your thumb and the side of the bent index finger of your right hand stroke down the Achilles tendon from where the tendon appears from the calf muscle down to the heel.

- Repeat 5 times.

Intention

To warm and loosen the Achilles tendon and continue to loosen the ankle joint in order to encourage the flow of energy in this area.

27 ~ Knuckle Across Sen Sahatsarangsi/Thawari on the Top of the Foot

Sen Line – Shatsarangsi/Thawari.
Reflex Points – Diaphragm.

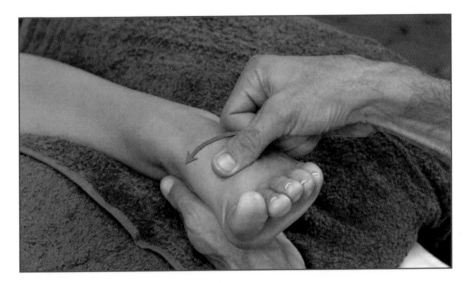

How to...

- Hold the foot in your left hand and then using your right hand make a loose fist.

- Using the second knuckle of all the fingers on your right hand press and drag your knuckles across the dorsum of the foot in a straight line from the highest point nearest the medial edge out to the lateral edge.

- Work along this line (about a quarter of the way down the Dorsum of the foot between the hollow at the top of the foot and the beginning of the toes).

- Repeat 10 times.

Intention

To relax the diaphragm muscle and assist deep relaxed breathing.

28 ~ Thumb Slide Down in Front of and then Around Ankle – one side then other

Sen Line – Sahatsarangsi/Thawari and Kalathari (medially). Ittha/Pingkala and Kalathari (laterally).

Reflex Points – Lymphatic system (lower body), hip joint, uterus or prostate, rectum and anus (medially). Hip joint, sexual organs, lower abdomen, and lymphatic system (upper body) (laterally).

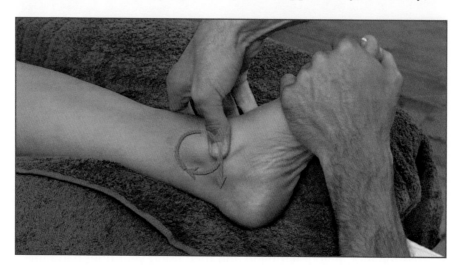

How to...

- Starting on the inside (medial side) of the ankle, hold the foot in your left hand, and with your right hand held open place the hand on the top (dorsum) of the foot so that your fingers are pointing toward the outside of the ankle and your thumb is pointing towards the inside of the ankle.

- Slide your thumb down just below the ankle, slide back up and repeat 10 times.

- Use the movement of your whole hand and wrist to help the movement.

- On the last slide down continue the movement of the thumb around the ankle so that your thumb circles under the ankle, over the tibia, around the top of the ankle and back to where you started.

- Repeat 10 times.

• Repeat both moves on the outside of the ankle, with the left hand.

Intention

To stimulate the lymphatic system of the lower and upper body and relax the hip joint before encouraging the flow of energy from the base of the spine.

29 ~ Knuckle Slide Along the Channels on the Top of the Foot

Sen Line – Kalathari.
Reflex Points – Lymphatic system, ribs, diaphragm, larynx trachea and vocal chords, labyrinth (inner ear) and chest.

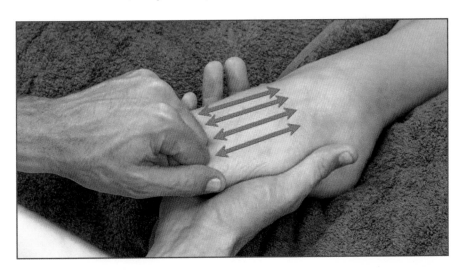

How to...

• Hold the sole of the foot in the palm of your right hand.

• Make a loose fist with your left hand and place the loose fist on the top of the dorsum near to the ankle joint, so that the second knuckle of each finger is resting in a channel on the top of the foot.

• Stroke the knuckles down the channels on the dorsum of the foot from the ankle to the toes.

• Repeat 10 times.

The Opening Sequence

Intention

To further relax your client emotionally, encourage deeper breathing, and further stimulate the lymphatic system of the upper body. Clearing the way for a free flow of energy through the chest area and upwards.

30 ~ Spiral Knuckle Top of Foot, Medial Arch and Both Sides of the Heel

Sen Line – Sumana, Ittha/Pingkala, Kalathari.

Reflex Points – Groin, lymphatic system, ribs, diaphragm, larynx trachea and vocal chords, labyrinth (inner ear), chest (top of foot). Cervical, thoracic, lumbar and sacral vertebrae and coccyx, penis or vagina, bladder, parathyroid (Medial arch). Coccyx, sexual organs, uterus or prostate (heel).

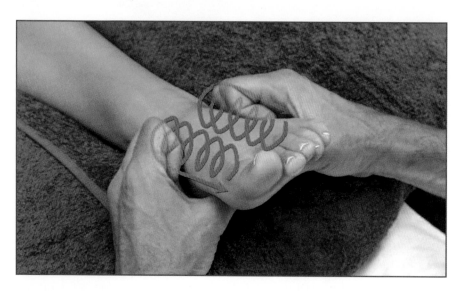

How to...

- Clench the fingers of both hands loosely. Place your thumbs on the sole of the foot near to the toes and rest the distal knuckles of your right hand on the dorsum of the foot, and the distal knuckles of your left hand on the medial arch of the foot.

- Circle the knuckles towards you and the midline of the foot, and then away from you and towards the inside and outside edge of the foot to create a circular movement with each hand.

- Move the hand from the wrist to create the movement

- As you circle move the hands along the foot towards the heel so that the circles become spirals.

- Finish at the heel so that you are circling the knuckles on both the inside and outside of the heel.

- Spiral knuckle back up and then down 5 times.

Intention

To further relax the spine and encourage the lymphatic system in the upper body and the flow of energy from the foot and up through the body.

31 ~ Press Points in the Channels on Top of the Foot

Sen Line – Kalathari.

Reflex Points – Thoracic lymph nodes, larynx trachea and vocal chords, labyrinth (inner ear).

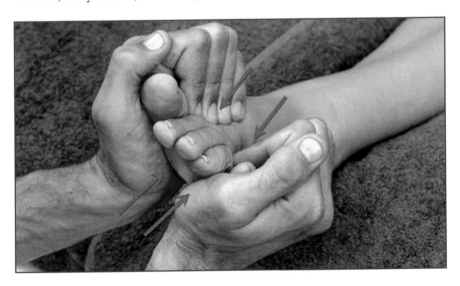

How to…

- Hold your hands together in the prayer position, and then open your hands and fingers whilst keeping the wrists together so that your hand resembles a lotus flower.

- Hold the foot in the palms of both hands and then bend the fingers so that fingers of the left hand press into the channel between the big toe and the next toe, and the fingers of your right hand press into the channel between little toe and the fourth toe.

- Press with your fingers, squeezing the channel between the pads of the fingers and the palm of your hand.

- Hold and press as you rock forwards and release as you rock back and then repeat 3 times.

Intention

To help to physically and emotionally balance your partner whilst working with the lymphatic system of the chest.

---

32 ~ Thumb Slide Up and Down the Channels on Top of the Foot

Sen Line – Kalathari.

Reflex Points – Groin, lymph system, ribs, diaphragm, larynx trachea and vocal chords, labyrinth (inner ear), chest.

How to…

- Hold the foot with both hands, with your fingers on the sole of the foot and your thumbs on the dorsum of the foot.

- Place your thumbs either side of the middle toe next to the first knuckle where the toe joins the foot.

- You will feel the start of a channel between the tendons that continues up to the hollow at the top of the foot, where the foot joins the leg.

- Now slide your thumbs up these two channels either side of the middle toe, up to the hollow where the foot joins the leg, and then slide the

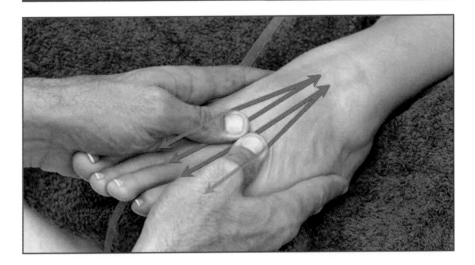

thumbs back down the two other channels between the toes so that your right thumb finishes between the fourth toe and little toe and your left thumb finishes between the big toe and second toe.

- Now repeat the thumb slides, but in reverse so that you slide up to the hollow from the two outside channels and then back down the two inside channels to where you started from.

- Repeat 10 times.

Intention

Emotional and physical balance as well as stimulating the entire lymphatic system.

33 ~ Thumb Slide Around Ankles

Sen Line – Sumana, Kalathari, Ittha/Pingkala, Sahatsarangsi/ Thawari.
Reflex Points – Chest, thoracic lymph nodes, diaphragm, ribs, hip joint, uterus or prostate, sexual organs, rectum and anus, lower abdomen.

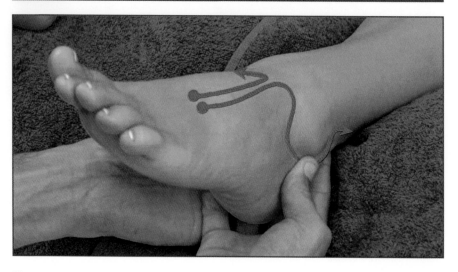

How to...

- Keep your hands as before, fingers on the sole and thumbs on the dorsum of the foot.

- Start midway along the two central channels on the dorsum of the foot and thumb slide up to the centre of the hollow where the foot joins the leg. It should feel as if there is a soft spot here.

- Without breaking the flow of the movement of your thumbs, move your fingers behind the heel of the foot and continue to slide your thumbs under the ankle (right thumb to the outside and left thumb to the inside of the ankle) and off the Achilles tendon.

- Repeat 10 times.

Intention

Further relaxing of the ankle joint enabling better energy flow along with more relaxing of the lower abdominal area and internal organs.

The Opening Sequence

34 ~ Thumbs Criss Cross Along the Top of the Foot

Sen Line – Kalathari.
Reflex Points – Groin, lymphatic system, ribs, diaphragm, larynx trachea and vocal chords, labyrinth (inner ear), chest.

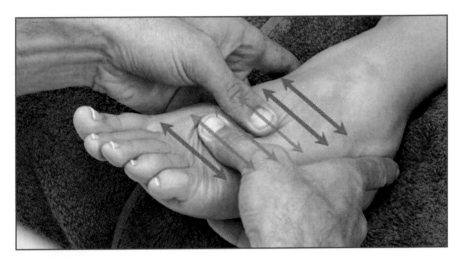

How to...

- Still with the fingers on the sole of the foot and the thumbs on the dorsum.

- Starting with your thumbs on the dorsum near to the toes, slide your right thumb from the lateral edge of the foot towards the medial edge of the foot so that it slides across the channels.

- At the same time slide your left thumb across the channels from the medial edge towards the lateral edge so that they cross over each other, one slightly higher than the other (it does not matter which one).

- Now slide both thumbs back to where they started.

- Move both thumbs slightly higher up the foot (toward the ankle) and repeat, but change whichever thumb was higher up the foot so that this time the other thumb is higher.

- Continue this criss-cross thumb slide all the way up the dorsum of the foot and over the hollow where the foot joins the leg.

- Criss-cross thumb slide back down to the toes and repeat 5 times.

- Finish this thumb slide at the hollow of the foot.

Intention

With the channels of Sen Kalathari in mind we are still aiming to relax the mind and emotions of our client and encourage the flow of energy from the foot throughout the body. The technique employed here is good for encouraging the flow of stagnant energy.

35 ~ Alternate Thumb Slide over the Hollow at the Top of the Foot

Sen Line – Sahatsarangsi/Thawari.

Reflex Points – Groin, lymphatic system (upper and lower body).

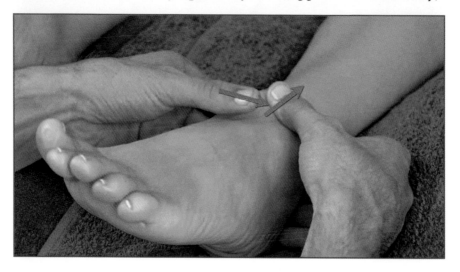

How to...

- Continuing on from the previous movement thumb slide the right thumb up over the hollow at the top of the foot and along the lateral edge of the tibia, and then repeat with the left thumb.

- Continue this alternate thumb slide many times.

Intention

To encourage further relaxation of the ankle joint and encourage the energy flow from the lower abdominal and groin area.

36 ~ Knuckle Slide Across the Balls of the Toes

Sen Line – Kalathari.
Reflex Points – Shoulder, lung, trapezius, thyroid, oesophagus, ear, eye.

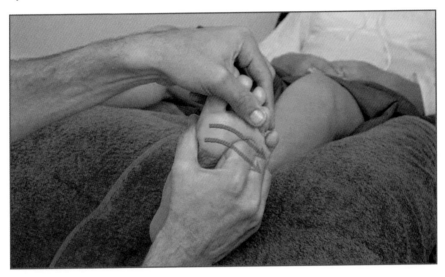

How to...

- Hold the foot with your left hand and press the foot back slightly so that the sole of the foot is more visible and accessible.

- Put your fingers on the dorsum and the thumb on the bottom of the foot near to the base of the toes so that the toes are also pressed back slightly.

- Make a fist with your right hand and slide the second knuckle of all the fingers across the balls of the toes with some pressure.

- Use your thumb on the medial edge of the foot as an anchor for this move.

- Repeat 10 times.

Intention

To deeply warm up the foot in preparation for the next section and to enable the flow of energy through the upper body towards the head.

The Opening Sequence

37 ~ Knuckle Slide Down and then Up the Sole of the Foot

Sen Line – Kalathari.

Reflex Points – Solar plexus, adrenal, kidney, stomach, pancreas, duodenum, heart (left), liver (right), spleen (left), gall bladder (right), ureter, transverse colon, small intestines, descending colon (left), ascending colon (right), rectum and anus (left), insomnia point.

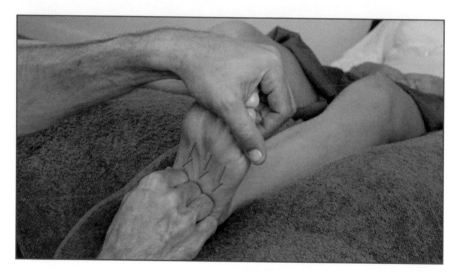

How to…

- Continue to hold the foot as for the previous technique.

- Slide the knuckles of the right hand down the sole of the foot from the balls of the toes to the heel as you rock forwards.

- Repeat 10 times.

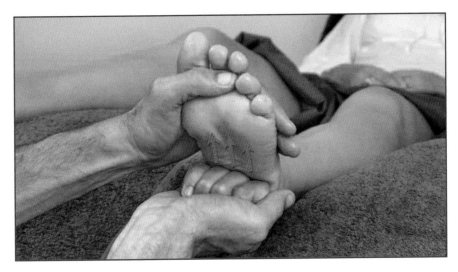

- Continue to hold the foot in your left hand, but don't press the foot back.
- Turn you right hand up and slide the knuckles of the right hand up the sole of the foot from the heel to the balls of the toes as you rock backwards.
- Repeat 10 times.

Intention

To deeply warm up the sole of the foot in preparation for the next section and to stimulate all the internal organs.

This concludes the warm-up section. If this is early on in your practice I would advise repeating this section on the other foot. If you feel confident with this section continue onto the next section working on the same foot.

The Reflex Points – Using the Stick

This section is mainly about working the reflex points with the stick in order to stimulate the internal organs. Whilst it is possible to use the stick to create a greater depth of pressure it has also been designed as a tool to save your knuckles. It is our intention to use it for the latter purpose and keep the pressure comfortable for your client. If you have no stick then you can use the first knuckle of your index finger or the blunt end of a pencil.

As well as working the reflex points with the stick, there are also some massage techniques performed with the stick prior to working the reflex points.

Holding a Massage Stick

There are various ways to hold a Thai Foot Massage stick, and whilst it may seem strange at first it becomes very natural very quickly. The following are the most common techniques for holding, and working with a stick:

- *Pen Holding Technique* – hold the stick like a pen! This is quite a gentle technique. You have to try quite hard to get a deeper pressure. It is great to begin with as most people still remember how to hold a pen.

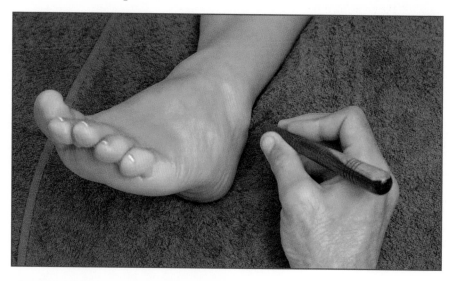

The Reflex Points ~ Using the Stick

- *Knife Holding Technique* – Hold the stick in the palm of your hand and extend your index finger to create some pressure. This is again a simple and relatively gentle technique.

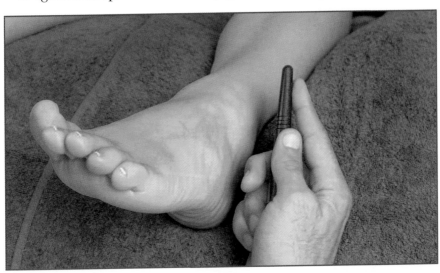

- *Thumbs Up Technique* – extend your thumb along the stick so that you can apply pressure with the stick using your thumb. This can be quite a strong technique and uses the weight of your arm to create the pressure.

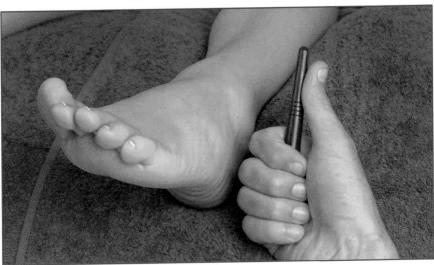

- *Extension of Arm Technique* – Hold the end of the stick in the centre of the palm of your hand and close all your fingers around the shaft of the stick. You can then use the weight of your arm to apply pressure through the stick. This is quite a strong technique.

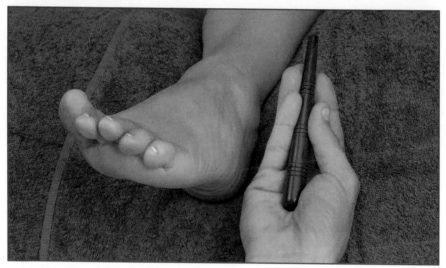

Reinforcing with the other thumb – With all of these techniques it is possible to use the free thumb to reinforce the technique and make it stronger. To do this you hold the stick in your preferred technique and apply some pressure as normal, then use the other thumb to increase the pressure by also pressing on the stick near to the tip.

Massaging With the Stick

38 ~ Apply the Cream to the Top of the Foot

Sen Line – Kalathari.
Reflex Points – Thoracic lymph nodes, chest, larynx trachea and vocal chords, labyrinth (inner ear).

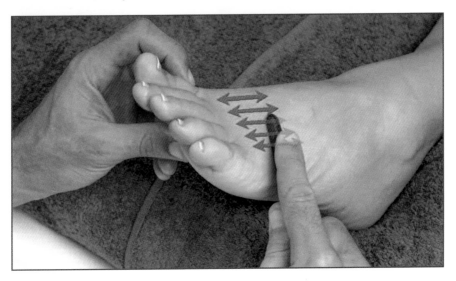

How to...

- Hold the stick as you would a knife, with your index finger extended along the blade.

- Apply some cream to the stick and rub this cream over the dorsum of the foot. Only apply the cream to the half of the dorsum near the toes.

Intention

To lubricate the foot for the next technique.

39 ~ Slide the Channels and Press with the Stick

Sen Line – Kalathari.

Reflex Points – Lymph glands (chest), larynx, trachea and vocal chords, labyrinth (inner ear), chest.

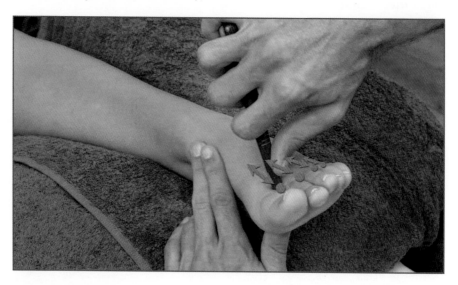

How to

- Now hold the thick end of the stick in your fist with your thumb extended towards the thin end of the stick.

- Bring your fist over the dorsum of the foot with your thumb and the thin end of the stick pointing towards you.

- Using your thumb as a guide, slide the thin end of the stick up and down the top half of the channel between the big toe and the second toe. Only work along the half of the dorsum nearest the toes, where the channels are more obvious.

- Repeat this stick slide up and down 10 times and then apply a steadily increasing then decreasing pressure at the tip of the channel between the knuckles of the toes. Raise your elbow and apply pressure to the stick using your thumb.

- Now repeat for all four channels, sliding the stick up and down ten times and then applying 5–10 seconds of pressure at the end of the channel.

Intention

Deeply stimulate the reflex points covered and initiate energy flow
along Sen Kalathari.

40 ~ Stick Slide the Medial Arch of the Foot

Sen Line – Sumana.
Reflex Points – Cervical, thoracic, lumbar and sacral vertebrae and
coccyx, penis or vagina, bladder, parathyroid.

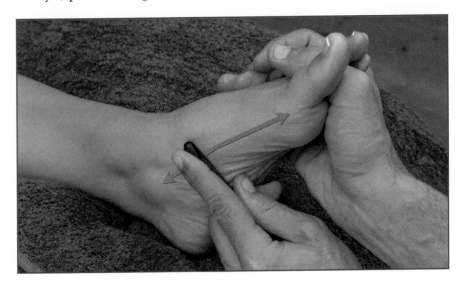

How to...

- Hold the stick in your left hand using the knife holding technique and
  hold the lateral edge of the foot in your right hand.

- Using your index finger as a guide slide the stick along the medial arch
  of the foot from big toe to heel.

- Repeat 10 times.

Intention

To relax the limbs and encourage a free flow of energy throughout
these areas and towards the body.

41 ~ Stick Slide the Lateral Arch of the Foot

Sen Line – Ittha/Pingkala.
Reflex Points – Shoulder, arm, elbow, knee.

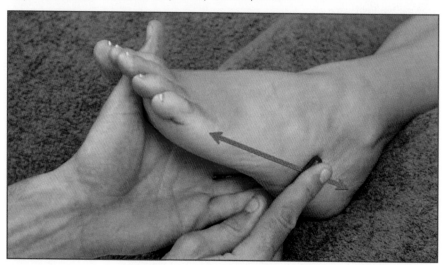

How to...

- Repeat the previous move, but this time work on the lateral edge of the foot, holding the stick in your right hand and the foot in your left hand.

Intention

To relax the spine and encourage the awakening and free flow of energy from the base of the spine.

42 ~ Stick Slide Sides of Toes and Twist in the Webbing

Sen Line – Kalathari, Ittha/Pingkala, Sumana.
Reflex Points – Sinuses.

How to...

- Hold the foot in your left hand near to the base of the toes. If the clients foot is larger than your hand you may prefer to hold each toe individually.

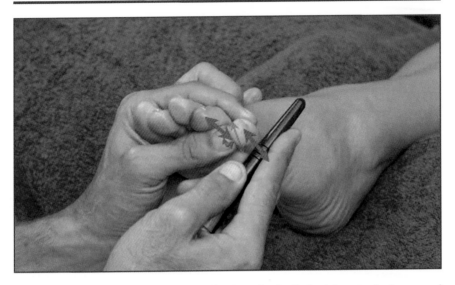

- Hold the stick in your right hand using the knife holding technique and use your index finger as a guide as you slide the stick up and down the lateral edge of the little toe 10 times.

- Now using your left hand gently spread the toes so that you can work between the little toe and the fourth toe.

- Slide the stick up and down the medial edge of the little toe 10 times.

- Keeping the toes spread apart use the edge of the stick on the webbing between the toes.

- Hold the stick against the webbing and then twist the stick on the webbing by rotating your wrist 10 times.

- Now repeat by sliding the stick on both the lateral edge and the medial edge of the fourth toe and then twist the stick in the webbing.

- Repeat so that both the medial and lateral edge of each toe is worked and the webbing between each toe is worked.

- Finish on the medial edge of the big toe.

Intention

This technique is used to clear the sinuses and encourage easy breathing whilst releasing stagnant energy from the head.

43 ~ Stick Press and Flick off the Tip of the Toes

Sen Line – Kalathari.
Reflex Points – Brain.

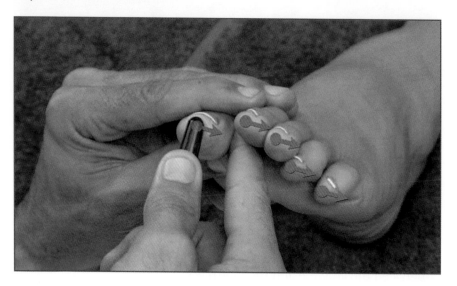

How to...

- Hold the stick in a loose fist in your right hand so that the fingers are supporting the stick. Extend your thumb along the stick towards the tip.

- Extend your index finger to the lateral edge of the big toe to stabilise this technique.

- Use your thumb on the side of the stick near to the tip to apply a steadily increasing pressure with the tip of the stick to the tip of the big toe.

- Allow this pressure to build and then let the stick flick or slide off of the big toe laterally, so that it comes to rest on the edge of your extended index finger.

- This is quite a hard technique to perform, however with some practice it becomes second nature, and can be performed quite quickly.

- Repeat 10 times on the tip of each toe, starting with the big toe and ending with the little toe.

Intention

This works the very tip of the toes and stimulates Sen Kalathari, and the brain. The intended effect is to stimulate the brain whilst relaxing the emotions.

44 ~ Stick Slide the Base of the Toes

Sen Line – Kalathari.
Reflex Points – Ear, eye, neck/throat.

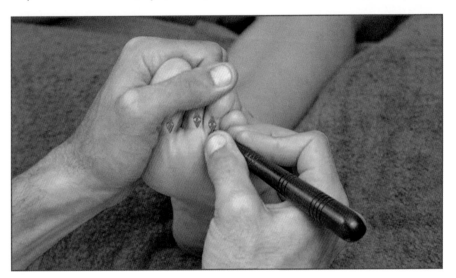

How to...

- Hold the stick like a pen and draw a line with the stick down the toes from just below the second knuckle of the toe to the base of the toe.

- Repeat this 10 times for each toe.

Intention

This technique encourages the flow of energy to the left side of the head (when working on the left foot), specifically the neck and throat, left ear and left eye.

45 ~ Stick Side Across the Ball of the Toes

Sen Line – Kalathari.
Reflex Points – Oesophagus, thyroid, lung, trapezius, ear, eye, shoulder.

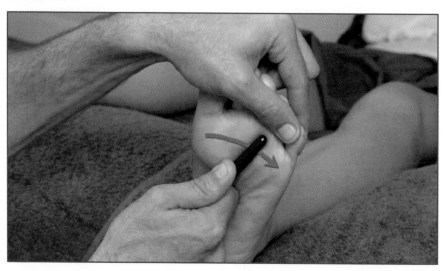

How to...

- Hold the stick in the fist of your right hand with your thumb extended towards the tip of the stick.

- Place your fist against the sole of the foot and use your thumb to press the side of the stick against the ball of the big toe.

- Rotate your fist in a clockwise direction in the centre of the sole of the foot, and press your thumb against the stick so that there is some pressure applied to the balls of all of the toes with the side of the stick as the stick slides across the balls of the toes.

- Slide the stick across the balls of the toes from the big toe to the little toe and repeat 10 times.

Intention

This technique relaxes the whole of the thoracic area to the front, back and sides of the body. Emotional tension is often held in the trapezius and shoulder area. The working of these reflex points and Sen Kalathari will help to release emotional tension.

The Reflex Points ~ Using the Stick

46 ~ Stick Slide Around the Ball of the Big Toe

Sen Line – Kalathari.
Reflex Points – Thyroid gland.

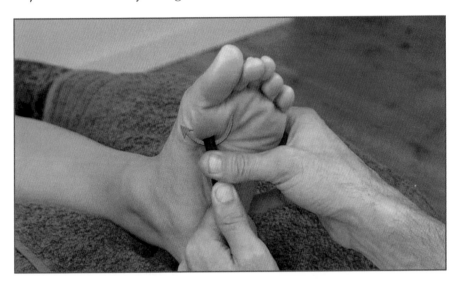

How to...

- Hold the stick in your left hand and touch the thin end of the stick against the balls of the toes, between the ball of the big toe and the second toe.

- Place the fingers of your right hand on the dorsum of the foot to steady it and use the thumb of your right hand to guide and press the stick down and around the ball of the big toe.

- Start near to the webbing between the big toe and the second toe and work around to the medial arch below the ball of the big toe.

- Repeat 10 times.

Intention

This technique is intended to stimulate the thyroid gland and optimise and stabilise the metabolic rate of the body.

47 ~ Stick Slide 3 Lines Down the Sole of the Foot

Sen Line – Kalathari.

Reflex Points – Lung, shoulder, heart and spleen (left), liver (right), descending colon (left), ascending colon (right) (lateral line). Lung, adrenal, solar plexus, kidney, transverse colon, small intestine, rectum (left), insomnia point, sexual organs (Mid Line). Thyroid, stomach, pancreas, duodenum, transverse colon, small intestine, urinary bladder, anus (left) (Medial Line).

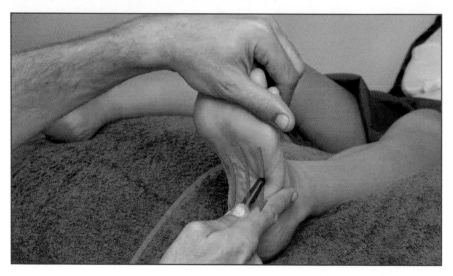

How to...

- Hold the stick in your right hand in a loose fist. Touch the thin end of the stick against the sole of the foot, just below the ball of the little toe.

- Whilst holding the foot with your left hand, slide the stick down from the ball of the little toe to the start of the heel.

- Repeat this stick slide down the centre line (starting below the ball of the middle toe to the start of the heel) and again for the medial line (starting below the ball of the big toe to the start of the heel).

- You can use the index finger of your right hand along the lateral edge of the foot as a guide for the lateral and central lines, and the thumb of your left hand on the stick as a guide for the medial line.

- Repeat 5 times for each line.

The Reflex Points ~ Using the Stick

NB: This technique can feel quite sensitive. A less intense alternative is to use the thick end of the stick

---

Intention

This technique stimulates many reflex points individually with a general technique.

---

48 ~ Criss Cross the Sole of the Foot with the Stick

Sen Line – Kalathari, Sahatsarangsi/Thawari.

Reflex Points – Sexual organs, insomnia point, large intestine, small intestine, bladder, kidney, ureter, pancreas, stomach, duodenum, solar plexus, shoulder, lung, thyroid, adrenal, heart (left), spleen (left), liver (right), gall bladder (right).

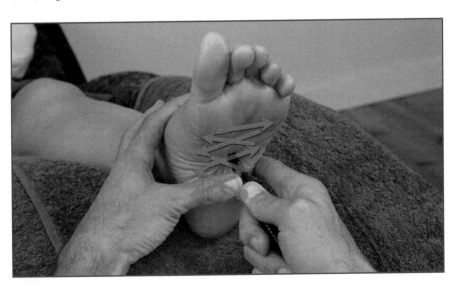

How to...

- Using the thin end of the stick, zig zag up the sole of the foot from the heel to the balls of the toes.

- At the balls of the toes slide the thin end of the stick across to the other edge of the foot and zig zag the stick back down to the heel of the foot.

The Reflex Points ~ Using the Stick

- Use your left hand to support the foot around the medial arch and your right hand on the stick.

- The thumb of your left hand can be used to support the stick and help with this movement.

> **Intention**
>
> As with the last technique this one also stimulates many internal organs via their reflex points, and again stimulates each point individually, within a general movement of the stick

49 ~ Stick Slide Up and Down the Sole of the Foot using the Side of the Stick

Sen Line – Kalathari.

Reflex Points – Insomnia point, large intestine, small intestine, bladder, kidney, ureter, pancreas, stomach, duodenum, solar plexus, shoulder, thyroid, adrenal, heart (left), spleen (left), liver (right), gall bladder (right).

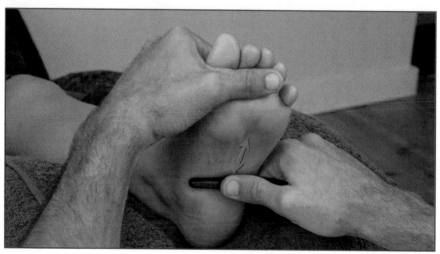

How to...

- Hold the stick in your right fist with your thumb extended along the stick towards the tip.

- Place the side of the stick against the sole of the foot, using your right thumb to create some depth of pressure.

- Now slide the side of the stick up and down the sole of the foot so that the stick covers the whole of the sole of the foot.

- Gently rock backwards as you slide the stick up towards the balls of the toes and rock forwards as you slide the stick back down the sole of the foot towards the heel.

- You will find that you apply more pressure as you rock forwards and down the sole of the foot, but still keep the stick in contact with the foot as you rock backwards and slide back up.

- Repeat 10 times.

Intention

To generally stimulate the internal organs via their reflex points. This technique is quite soothing after the two previous techniques.

50 ~ Stick Slide Across the Top of the Heel

Sen Line – Kalathari, Sahatsarangsi/Thawari.
Reflex Points – Bladder, rectum and anus (left), small intestine, descending colon (left), ascending colon (right).

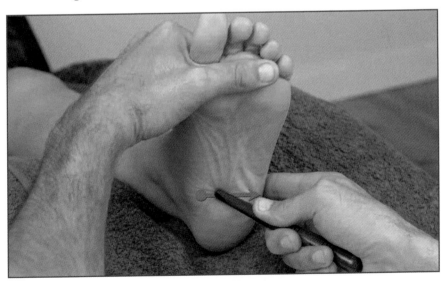

How to...

- Holding the stick in your right fist with the thumb extended towards the tip. Hold the top of the foot in your left hand.

- Touch the tip of the stick on the medial arch, at the top of the heel.

- Extend your index finger to the lateral edge of the foot at the top of the heel.

- Increase the pressure by squeezing your index finger and thumb towards each other, pressing the stick more firmly onto the foot.

- As this pressure begins to increase slide the tip of the stick across the top of the heel from the medial edge to the lateral edge.

- Repeat from the start 10 times.

Intention

To promote elimination via the bladder and colon.

51 ~ Stick Slide Down on the Heel

Sen Line – Kalathari, Sahatsarangsi/Thawari.
Reflex Points – Sexual organs, insomnia point, sciatic nerve.

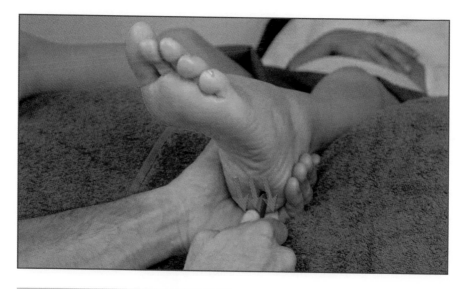

The Reflex Points ~ Using the Stick

How to...

- Hold the stick in your right hand as if you were passing a knife to someone.

- Imagine you have drawn a line across the top of the heel in the previous move (it may not be too hard to imagine). Now touch the tip of the stick (thin end) at any point along this line.

- Apply some pressure and then slide the stick straight down to the bottom of the heel of the foot.

- Now repeat the same technique 10 times, each time starting from a different point along the "line" at the top of the heel.

- You can support the heel of the foot in your left hand, which will raise the foot slightly so that it is easier for you to slide off the heel with the stick.

> **Intention**
>
> Deep stimulation of the reflex points.

52 ~ Hack the Heel with the Thick End of the Stick

Sen Line – Kalathari.
Reflex Points – Sexual organs, insomnia point, sciatic nerve.

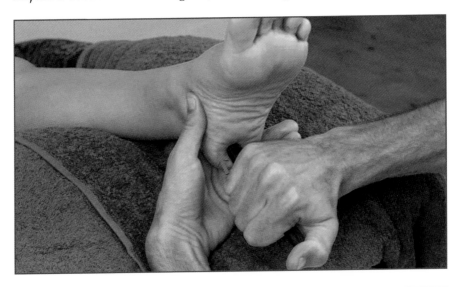

How to...

- Hold the stick tightly in you fist, and turn your hand so that the back of the hand is uppermost.

- Now bring your hand towards your body by bending the arm at the elbow.

- Bring your elbow wide so that the thick end of the stick is now pointing toward the heel of the foot and the thin end of the stick is pointing to you.

- Hit the heel of the foot with the thick end of the stick and repeat many times covering the whole of the heel of the foot.

- Only hit the heel of the foot.

Intention

Further stimulation of these reflex points and a shifting of energy up through the body.

Stimulating the Reflex Points

Now dry the foot, stick and your hands to remove the cream. Using cream for this section makes it harder to work the points as the stick may slip, to avoid this the cream is removed.

Work around the points shown on the diagram below starting at number 1. Use whichever stick holding technique feels most appropriate, and experiment with the way you hold the stick until you feel comfortable. Apply a gradually increasing and then gradually decreasing pressures as you rock forwards and then back. There should be a brief pause at the end of your rock forwards to hold the pressure momentarily. Try rocking forward for 3 seconds, pausing for 1, and rocking back for 3.

Use your free hand to support the foot near to the point that you are working so that if you slip with the stick you slip into your own finger and not your clients foot.

The Reflex Points ~ Using the Stick

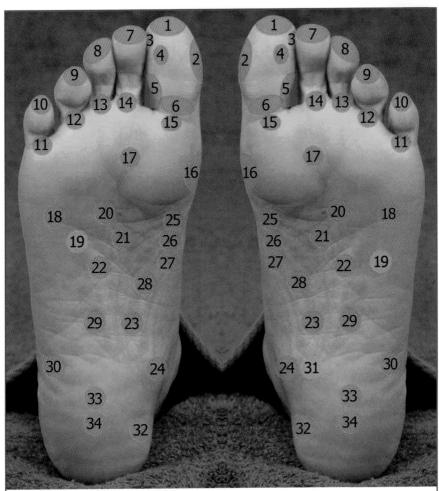

1 Frontal Sinuses	14 Eyes	25 Stomach
2 Nose	15 Hypertension Point	26 Pancreas
3 Temples	16 Parathyroid Gland	27 Duodenum
4 Pituitary Gland	17 Thyroid Gland	28 Transverse Colon
5 Brain Stem	18 Heart (left) Liver	29 Small Intestine
6 Neck/Throat	(right)	30 Descending Colon
7 Frontal Sinuses	19 Spleen (left) Gall	(left) Caecum/
8 Frontal Sinuses	Bladder (right)	Appendix (right)
9 Frontal Sinuses	20 Solar Plexus	31 Rectum/Anus
10 Frontal Sinuses	21 Adrenal Gland	32 Sciatic Nerve
11 Ears	22 Kidney	33 Insomnia Point
12 Ears	23 Ureter	34 Sexual Organs
13 Eyes	24 Urinary Bladder	

Map showing the Reflex Points worked with the Stick

The Reflex Points ~ Using the Stick

This section offers a more focused and precise stimulation of the reflex points, however the technique is still general in its approach and aims to stimulate all the reflex points equally.

Now continue onto the third section
still working on the same leg.

Working the Sen Lines of the Leg

This section begins with a few techniques to warm the feet after the stick section, and then goes on to working the Sen lines of the legs. Having just worked the Reflex points this section encourages the energy released to flow throughout the body.

Finishing the Feet

53 ~ Apply Cream to Top and Bottom of the Foot (as for number 11)

Sen Line – Kalathari, Ittha/Pingkala, Sahatsarangsi/Thawari, Sumana.
Reflex Points – All superficially.

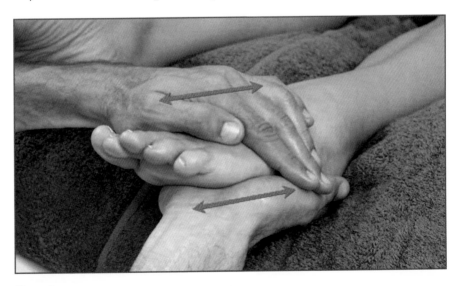

How to...

- Apply a scoop of cream to your hands, and warm the cream in your hands by circling the palms together.

- Clasp your hands together as if you have just clapped, or about to rub your palms together in glee!

- Then open your hands as you slide your fingers and then your palms down the foot, with one hand on top of the foot and the other on the sole of the foot.

- Stroke all the way down to the ankle and then slide back up with some pressure and release.

- Now turn the hands as if to clap with the other hand on top and repeat.

- Repeat and alternate many times.

Intention

To warm the foot in preparation for the next section.

54 ~ Thumb Slide Up and Down the Centre of the Sole of the Foot

Sen Line – Kalathari, Sahatsarangsi/Thawari.
Reflex Points – Lung, adrenal, solar plexus, kidney, transverse colon, ureter, small intestine, rectum and anus (left), insomnia point, sexual organs.

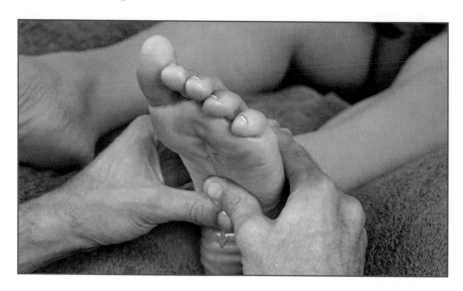

Working the Sen Lines of the Leg

How to...

- Place both of your thumbs along the centre line of the sole of the foot, just above the heel, with one thumb slightly higher than the other.
- Place the fingers of both hands on the dorsum of the foot for support.
- Slide both thumbs together, up and down the sole of the foot. From just above the heel of the foot to just below the ball of the middle toe.
- As you slide your thumbs up rock backwards and as you slide your thumbs down rock your body forwards.
- Repeat 10 times.

> **Intention**
>
> As well as encouraging the flow of energy from the foot, this technique also feels very soothing after working the reflex points with the stick.

55 ~ Thumb Slide Around the Ball of the Big Toe

Sen Line – Kalathari.
Reflex Points – Thyroid gland.

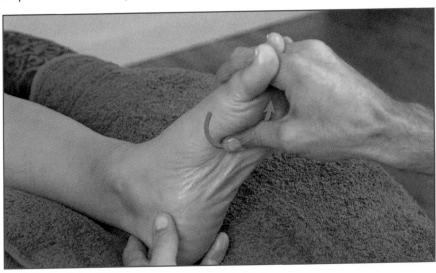

Working the Sen Lines of the Leg

How to…

- Place your index finger between the big toe and 2nd toe, your middle finger between the 2nd and 3rd toe, your ring finer between the 3rd and 4th toe and your little finger between the 4th and 5th toe, so that your finger tips are in each of the channels on the top of the foot.

- Now use the pad of your thumb to slide around the ball of the big toe.

- Start at the medial side of the big toe, slide down the medial edge, underneath the ball of the big toe and then back up towards your index finger between the balls of the big toe and 2nd toe.

- Repeat this 10 times.

Intention

To optimise the body's metabolic rate.

56 ~ Thumbs Criss Cross on the Sole of the Foot (as for number 15)

Sen Line – Kalathari, Sahatsarangsi/Thawari.

Reflex Points – Sexual organs, insomnia point, large intestine, small intestine, bladder, kidney, ureter, pancreas, stomach, duodenum, solar plexus, shoulder, lung, trapezius, thyroid, adrenal, heart (left), spleen (left), liver (right), gall bladder (right).

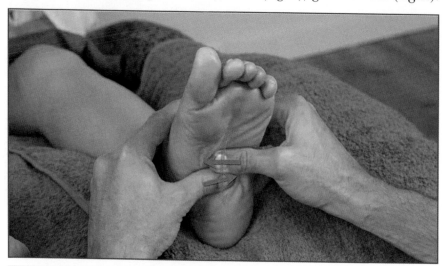

Working the Sen Lines of the Leg

How to...

- Starting at the centre of the heel with one thumb slightly higher than the other.

- Press in as you rock forward and slide the thumbs out to each side.

- Return your thumbs to the centre line a little higher than before, with the other thumb higher this time and repeat.

- Continue to the balls of the toes and then work back down to the heel

- Repeat 10 times.

> **Intention**
>
> A general and soothing technique for all of the reflex points on the sole of the foot.

57 ~ Thumb Slide Channels Two at a Time

Sen Line – Kalathari.
Reflex Points – Thoracic lymph nodes, larynx trachea and vocal chords, labyrinth (inner ear) chest.

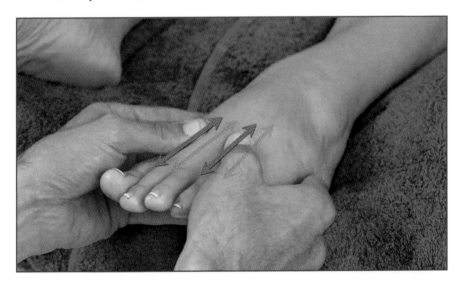

Working the Sen Lines of the Leg

How to…

- Place both thumbs on the top of the foot, with your fingers underneath the foot for support.

- Start with the thumbs in the channels on the top of the foot near to the toes.

- Slide both thumbs simultaneously up and down 2 of the channels 10 times. Don't work 2 channels next to each other as your thumbs may get in the way of each other.

- Only slide halfway up the dorsum of the foot, where the channel is most obvious.

- Now repeat the move in the other 2 channels on the top of the foot.

> **Intention**
>
> To clear the channels on top of the foot and allow energy to flow more freely.

58 ~ Thumb Pull in the Channels

Sen Line – Kalathari.

Reflex Points – Thoracic lymph nodes, larynx trachea and vocal chords, labyrinth (inner ear), chest.

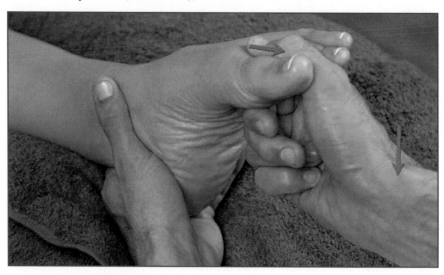

Working the Sen Lines of the Leg

How to…

- Hold your right hand as if you are passing a card to someone.

- Now lift your thumb, and place the thumb of your right hand on the top of the foot in the channel between the big toe and second toe.

- Your fingers should be below the foot in a loose fist, with your index finger underneath the channel that your thumb is on.

- Press your thumb into the channel (as if you have decided to hold on tightly to the card) and draw your thumb towards you so that your thumb slides up and off the channel.

- Repeat this once in each channel working from the big toe to the little toe.

Intention

To stimulate the energy along Sen Kalathari.

---

59 ~ Thumb Slide Up and Down the Channels on Top of the Foot (as for number 32)

Sen Line – Kalathari.
Reflex Points – Groin, lymphatic system, ribs, diaphragm, larynx trachea and vocal chords, labyrinth (inner ear), chest.

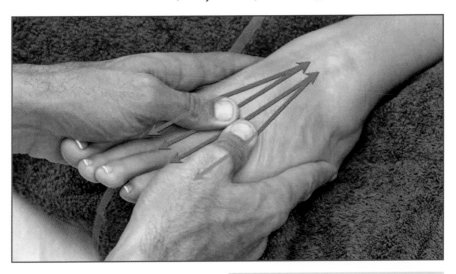

Working the Sen Lines of the Leg

How to...

- Hold the foot with both hands, with your fingers on the sole of the foot and your thumbs on the dorsum of the foot.

- Place your thumbs either side of the middle toe next to the first knuckle where the toe joins the foot.

- You will feel the start of a channel between the tendons that continues up to the hollow at the top of the foot, where the foot joins the leg.

- Now slide your thumbs up these two channels either side of the middle toe, up to the hollow where the foot joins the leg, and then slide the thumbs back down the two other channels between the toes so that your right thumb finishes between the fourth toe and little toe and your left thumb finishes between the big toe and second toe.

- Now repeat the thumb slides, but in reverse so that you slide up to the hollow from the two outside channels and then back down the two inside channels to where you started from

- Repeat 10 times.

Intention

Emotional and physical balance as well as stimulating the entire lymphatic system.

60 ~ Thumb Slide Around Ankles (as for number 33)

Sen Line – Sumana, Kalathari, Ittha/Pingkala, Sahatsarangsi/ Thawari.

Reflex Points – Chest, thoracic lymph nodes, diaphragm, ribs, hip joint, prostate or uterus, sexual organs, rectum and anus, lower abdomen.

How to...

- Keep your hands as before, fingers on the sole and thumbs on the dorsum of the foot.

Working the Sen Lines of the Leg

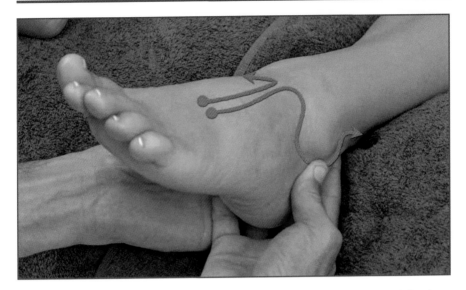

- Start midway along the two central channels on the dorsum of the foot and thumb slide up to the centre of the hollow where the foot joins the leg. You should feel a soft spot here.

- Without breaking the flow of movement of your thumbs, move your fingers to behind the heel of the foot and continue to slide your thumbs under the ankle (right thumb to the outside and left thumb to the inside of the ankle) and off the Achilles tendon.

- Repeat 10 times.

Intention

More relaxation of the abdominal area along with some lymphatic drainage.

61 ~ Thumbs Criss Cross on Hollow

Sen Line – Shatsarangsi/Thawari.
Reflex Points – Groin, lymphatic system (upper and lower body).

Working the Sen Lines of the Leg

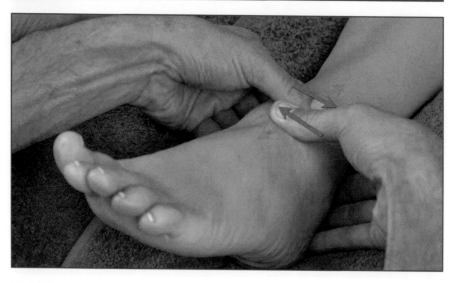

How to...

- Place both thumbs on the top of the foot, just below the hollow. So that your right thumb is pointing to the medial edge of the foot and your left thumb is pointing to the lateral edge of the foot.

- Place your fingers underneath the foot for support.

- Now slide your right thumb towards the medial edge and your left thumb towards the lateral edge so that they pass next to each other as they slide over the hollow.

- Now move whichever thumb was nearest to the toes, and place it next to the other thumb nearer to the leg, and repeat the thumb slide.

- Keep repeating this criss cross sequence up and down over the hollow at the top of the foot 10 times.

Intention

To encourage the energy to flow around the ankle joint and to stimulate the lymphatic system.

62 ~ Alternate Thumb Slide over the Hollow at the Top of the Foot (as for number 35)

Sen Line – Shatsarangsi/Thawari.
Reflex Points – Groin, lymphatic system (upper and lower body).

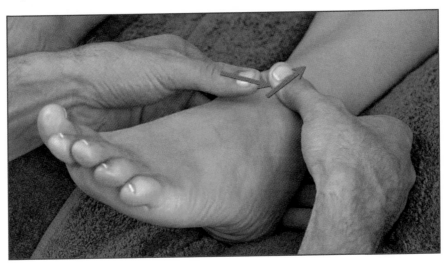

How to…

- Place both thumbs on the top of the foot, just below the hollow, as for the previous move.
- Slide the thumb, which is nearest the leg, so that it strokes over the hollow to the beginning of the leg.
- As the first thumb slides off at the leg, begin to slide the other thumb up over the hollow in the same manner.
- At the same time bring the first thumb back to its starting position, ready to slide over the hollow again.
- Keep repeating this alternate thumb slide at least 10 times.

Intention

To encourage deeper relaxation of the ankle joint and encourage the energy flow from the lower abdominal and groin area.

Working the Sen Lines of the Leg

63 ~ Knuckle the Big Toe

Sen Line – Kalathari.

Reflex Points – Mandible and maxilla.

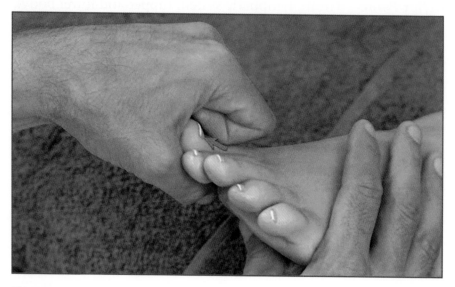

How to…

- Hook your index finger of your left hand and place the distal knuckle of the index finger on the top of the big toe between the knuckle of the big toe and the nail of the big toe.

- Hold the foot in your right hand for support.

- Using the distal knuckle of your index finger slide the knuckle up and down the area between the knuckle and the nail, as if you are scratching the area.

- Repeat this at least 10 times.

Intention

To release tension in the jaw.

Working the Sen Lines of the Leg

64 ~ Finger Slide Toes

Sen Line – Kalathari, Ittha/Pingkala, Sumana.

Reflex Points – Frontal sinuses, ear, eye. Big toe only – nose, neck/throat, temples, pituitary gland, brain stem, maxilla, mandible, tonsils.

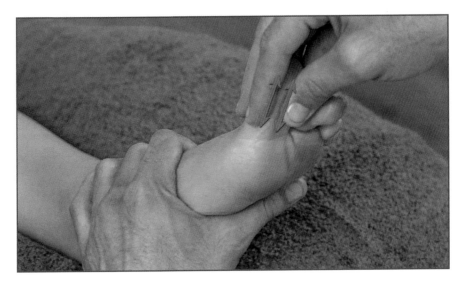

How to...

- Place the tips of all of the fingers of your right hand together, as if you are an Italian gesticulating, or so that your hand resembles a beak.

- Now place the tips of your fingers on the tip of the little toe.

- Let your fingers move apart slightly as you slide all of the fingers down the length of the toe and back up again.

- Repeat this 10 times.

- Your fingers should cover all sides of the toe if possible.

- Repeat this on each toe, finishing with the big toe.

Intention

Stimulates the frontal sinuses on all of the toes with additional stimulation of the head on the big toe.

65 ~ Click off the Toes

Sen Line – Kalathari.
Reflex Points – Sinuses and brain.

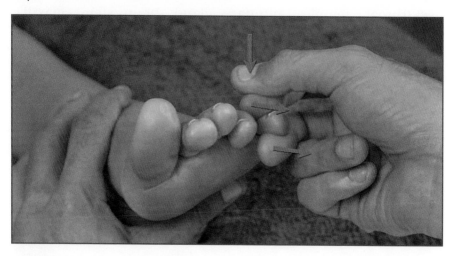

How to...

- Using your right hand, extend your first 2 fingers to resemble a pair of scissors.

- Now place the little toe between your extended fingers (at the end of the scissors)

- Bend your fingers so that you can place your thumb on top of the index finger

- Gently squeeze the tip of the toe between your thumb and fingers.

- When you have built up a gentle pressure, slide your fingers briskly off the toe so that your fingers snap together.

- There may be a snapping sound as your fingers click together, but this comes with practice and is not essential to the effectiveness of the move.

- Repeat this once for each toe.

Intention

This is the final stimulation of the reflex points on the foot before continuing onto the sen lines of the leg and finishes with the stimulation of the brain from the tips of the toes.

Working the Sen Lines of the Leg

Massaging the Leg Lines

Intention

The Intention for this whole section is to encourage the flow of energy that you have just awakened in the feet to flow throughout the body along the sen lines. The reflex points are not highlighted and are only touched upon in a few of the techniques.

66 ~ Apply Cream to the Outside of the Leg

Sen Line – Sahatsarangsi/Thawari, Ittha/Pingkala, Kalathari.

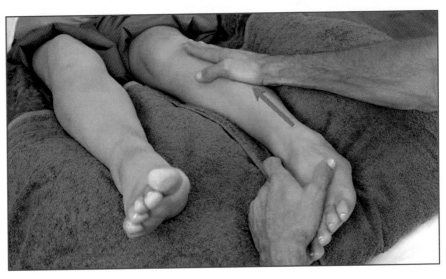

How to...

- Warm some cream in your hands as before, and apply the cream to the outside of the leg, using alternate hands.

- To begin with hold the foot in your right hand and turn the foot towards the midline so that the lateral side of the leg is more visible, and use your left hand to spread the cream on the outside of the leg. Then change hands, so that you are holding the foot with your left hand and spreading the cream with your right hand.

67 ~ Thumb Slide the Sen Lines on the Outside of the Leg

Sen Line – Sahatsarangsi/Thawari, Ittha/Pingkala, Kalathari.

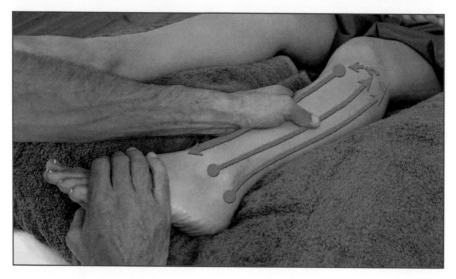

How to...

- Turn the foot towards the midline and hold the foot with your right hand.

- Using the thumb of your left hand just under the lateral ankle. Thumb slide up Sen Ittha/Pingkala, behind the ankle and along below the fibula to the top of the fibula. As you thumb slide up this line rock forwards.

- At the top of this line slide the thumb medially to the lateral edge of the tibia and slide down Sen Sahatsarangsi/Thawari, along the lateral edge of the tibia to the hollow at the top of the foot. As you thumb slide down this line rock backwards. Do not try to press with any force as you slide down this line.

- Now thumb slide up Sen Kalathari. Place the thumb of your left hand just above the lateral ankle and then thumb slide up the lower leg just above the fibula, to the top of the fibula. Rock forwards as you slide up this line and then rock backwards as you slide down Sen Sahatsarangsi/Thawari as before.

Working the Sen Lines of the Leg

- Repeat this technique of sliding up Sen Ittha/Pingkala, down Sen Sahatsarangsi/Thawari, up Sen Kalathari, and down Sahatsarangsi/Thawari between three to five times.

- Then thumb slide with alternate thumbs up Sen Sahatsarangsi/Thawari, from the hollow at the top of the foot, along the lateral edge of the tibia, to the top of the tibia.

68 ~ Apply Cream to the Inside of the Leg

Sen Line – Kalathari, Sahatsarangsi/Thawari.

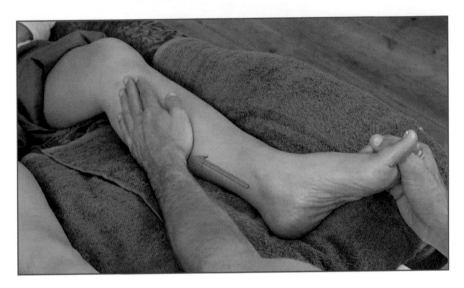

How to...

- Warm some cream in your hands and apply the cream as before, but this time to the inside of the lower leg.

- To begin with hold the foot in your left hand and turn the foot outwards so that the medial side of the leg is more visible. Then change hands, so that you are holding the foot with your right hand and spreading the cream with your left hand.

69 ~ Thumb Slide the Sen Lines on the Inside of the Leg

Sen Line – Sahatsarangsi/Thawari, Kalathari.

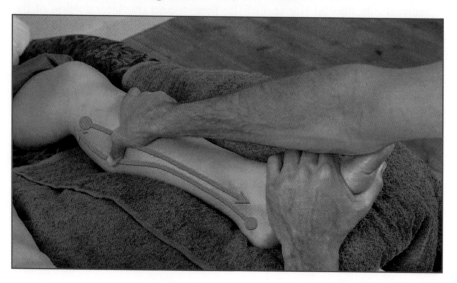

How to...

- Turn the foot laterally and hold the foot in your left hand.

- Using your right thumb, thumb slide up the inside of the lower leg along Sen Kalathari. Starting between the medial ankle and the Achilles tendon, up over the medial head of the calf muscle.

- Then slide the thumb slightly laterally and down Sen Sahatsarangsi/Thawari along the medial edge of the Tibia.

- Rock forwards as you thumb slide up Sen Kalathari and backwards as you slide down Sen Sahatsarangsi/Thawari. Repeat this three to five times.

- Then thumb slide with alternate thumbs up along Sen Sahatsarangsi/Thawari from just behind the medial ankle along the medial edge of the tibia to the top of the tibia.

Working the Sen Lines of the Leg

70 ~ Apply Cream to the Knee (medially to laterally)

Sen Line – Kalathari, Ittha/Pingkala, Sahatsarangsi/Thawari.

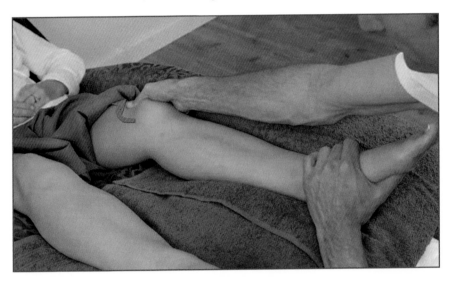

How to...

- Continue holding the foot with your left hand.

- Dip your right thumb in the cream and apply the cream to the area above the knee, towards the midline.

- Your right thumb now circles around the knee going up the medial edge of the knee and down the lateral edge of the knee.

- Your thumb however does not stay in contact with the leg for the entire circle. Instead the thumb is only in contact with the leg around the upper medial quarter around the knee.

- If you imagine a clock on the knee, you will just stroke around the knee, between 9 and 12 o'clock.

- By doing this circular movement you will create a nicer rhythm to the move, and be able to continue rocking your body forwards and backwards as you work.

- Repeat this 10 times.

Working the Sen Lines of the Leg

71 ~ Apply Cream to the Knee (laterally to medially)

Sen Line – Kalathari, Sahatsarangsi/Thawari.

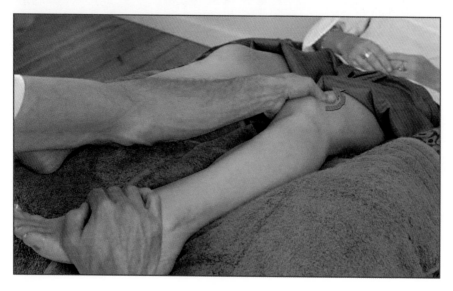

How to...

- Now change hands so that you are holding the foot towards the midline with your right hand.

- Use your left thumb this time, and using the same technique thumb stroke around the knee from between 3 and 12 o'clock.

- Repeat 10 times.

72 ~ Thumb Spiral Down the Outside of the Leg

Sen Line – Kalathari, Ittha/Pingkala, Sahatsarangsi/Thawari.

How to...

- Continue with your left thumb and spiral down the lateral edge of the leg.

- The previous move should flow into this move so that your left thumb continues to circle down the outside of the leg.

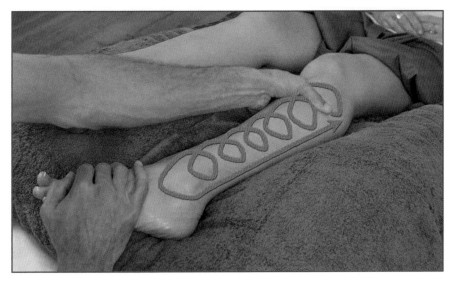

- Your thumb remains in contact with the leg for the complete spiral. The spiral goes in an anti-clockwise direction so that you are pushing up as you spiral down the leg.

- Make sure your spiral is large enough to cover all 3 outside lines.

- When you have spiralled down to the ankle, thumb spiral gently around the ankle and then slide the thumb up Sen Ittha/Pingkala then repeat the spiral down the outside of the leg.

- Repeat this technique 5 times.

73 ~ Thumb Spiral Down the Inside of the Leg

Sen Line – Kalathari, Sahatsarangsi/Thawari.

How to...

- Change hands and repeat the same technique on the inside of the leg to cover the 2 inside lines.

- Hold the foot in your left hand, and turn the foot outwards so that you can see the inside of the leg more easily.

Working the Sen Lines of the Leg

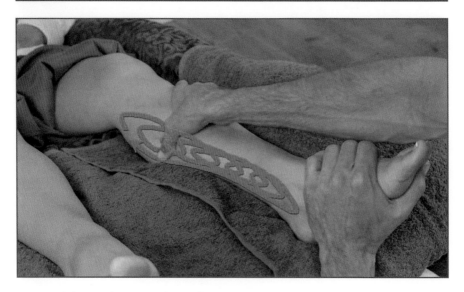

- Spiral down the 2 inside leg lines as for the previous move, so that you are pushing up as you spiral down.
- Repeat 5 times.

74 ~ Bend the Leg, support the Foot, and Massage the Knee

Sen Line – Sahatsarangsi/Thawari.

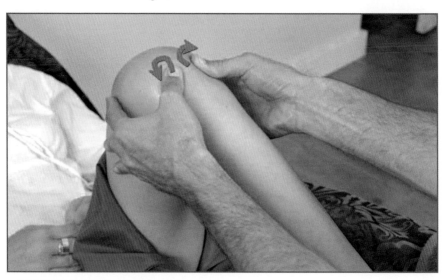

Working the Sen Lines of the Leg

How to…

- Place the palm of your right hand against the sole of the foot.

- Place your left hand underneath the knee.

- Now push against the sole of the foot, and as you do help the leg bend with your left hand by slightly lifting behind the knee.

- Continue to push the foot and bend the leg until the leg is bent to 90 degrees. The foot should now rest flat on the chair.

- As you bend the leg like this use more effort in pushing the foot as opposed to lifting the knee, otherwise it will be hard work.

- Support the foot, so that the leg stays where it is, without your client having to use any effort.

- Place both thumbs at the front of the knee, either side of the patella tendon. You should feel 2 soft points here.

- Gently press and rub here in small circular movements.

75 ~ Finger Slide Down the Back of the Leg

Sen Line – Sumana.

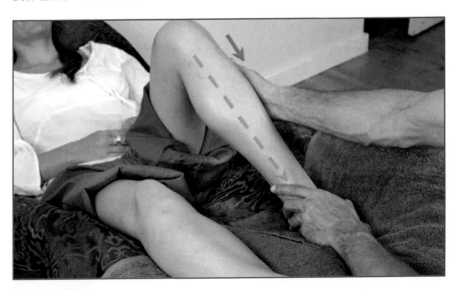

Working the Sen Lines of the Leg

How to...

- With one hand supporting the foot, slide the other hand from the front of the ankle up the lower leg to the knee.

- Now slide your hand behind the knee and, using the pads of your fingers, slide your fingers down the centre of the back of the lower leg to the ankle.

- Change hands and repeat so that one hand is always supporting the foot.

- As you slide your hand up the leg, rock your body forwards and, as you slide your hand down the back of the leg, rock your body backwards to create some pressure.

- You are working Sen Sumana here. You should feel that you are working between the 2 calf muscles at the back of the leg.

- You may need to apply more cream to the leg for this move and be aware of the pressure that you apply as this can be sensitive particularly half way down the leg.

- Repeat 5 times.

76 ~ Spiral Knuckle both Sides of the Leg

Sen Line – Kalathari, Ittha/Pingkala, Sahatsarangsi/Thawari.

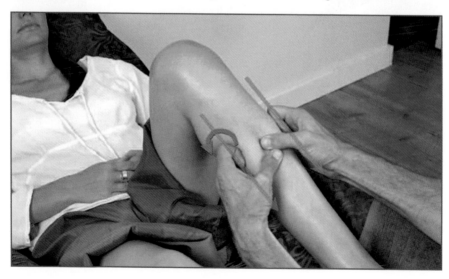

Working the Sen Lines of the Leg

How to...

- Support the foot so that the leg remains at rest.

- Place the thumbs of both hands on the front of the lower leg, and gently clench all of your fingers. So that the knuckles of the right hand are touching the muscle to the outside of the lower leg and the knuckles of the left hand are touching the muscle to the inside of the lower leg.

- Using the distal knuckles of all the fingers of both hands, spiral the knuckles away from you, downwards and then back and up towards you.

- Continue this spiralling movement all the way down the leg.

- Return to the top of the lower leg and repeat 5 times.

77 ~ Twist the Calf Laterally

Sen Line – Kalathari, Ittha/Pingkala, Sahatsarangsi/Thawari, Sumana.

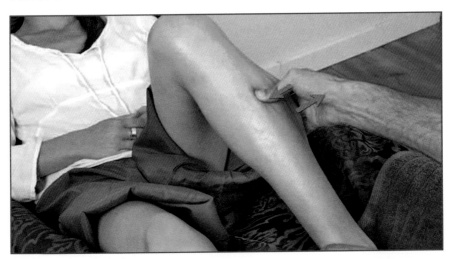

How to...

- Support the leg with your left hand, and use your right hand around the outside of the lower leg to draw the calf muscle towards you.

- Use the pads of the fingers of your right hand, between the calf muscles, along the centre line of the back of the lower leg.

- Start near to the knee and work your way down to the ankle.

- Lean your body backwards as you perform this technique and draw the calf muscle around the outside of the lower leg

- Sen Sahatsarangsi/Thawari can also be worked with the thumb of your right hand as you perform this technique. Try placing your thumb along Sen Sahatsarangsi/Thawari (along the lateral edge of the tibia or shinbone) and as you lean back turn your wrist towards the midline so that your thumb presses into Sen Sahatsarangsi/Thawari as you draw the calf muscle around the outside of the lower leg.

- This thumb press will not always be possible with big legs or little hands.

- Repeat 3–5 times.

78 ~ Slide up and Knuckle Slide Down the Outside of the Leg

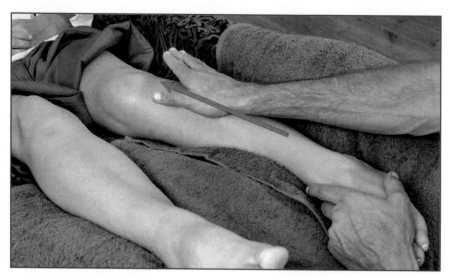

Sen Line – Kalathari, Ittha/Pingkala, Sahatsarangsi/Thawari.

Working the Sen Lines of the Leg

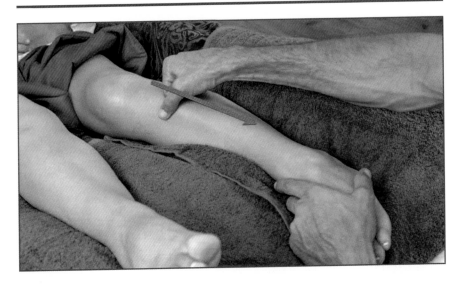

How to...

- Gently place the leg back down by supporting the knee as you lower the leg and by gently pulling the foot towards you.

- When the leg is placed back down use your left hand to turn and hold the foot gently towards the midline.

- With the heel of your right hand (the area on the palm of the hand next to the wrist) slide up the outside of the lower leg from just above the ankle to below the knee.

- Make sure you are not pressing onto bone as you do this, slide on the muscle between the Tibia and Fibula.

- At the top of this soft tissue near to the knee make a fist with your right hand and slide back down the lower leg, covering the same area with the second knuckle of all fingers.

- Repeat this 5 times.

79 ~ Slide up and Knuckle Slide Down the Inside of the Leg

Sen Line – Kalathari, Ittha/Pingkala, Sahatsarangsi/Thawari.

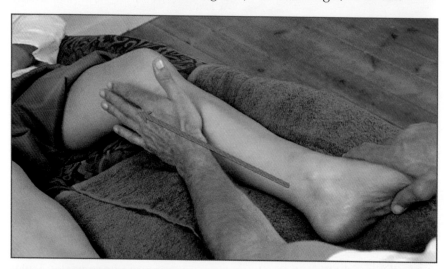

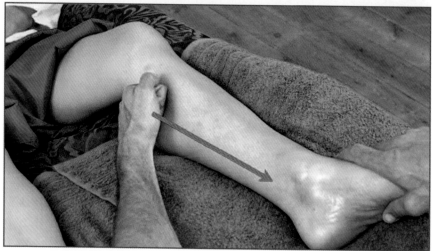

How to...

- Turn the foot and the leg laterally and hold the foot with your right hand.

- With the heel of your left hand (the area on the palm of the hand next to the wrist) slide up the inside of the lower leg from just above the ankle to below the knee.

Working the Sen Lines of the Leg

- Make sure you are not pressing onto bone as you do this, slide on the calf muscle below the Tibia.

- At the top of this soft tissue near to the knee, make a fist with your left hand and slide back down the lower leg, covering the same area, with the second knuckle of all fingers.

- Repeat this 5 times.

80 ~ Thumb Slide the Sen Lines on the Outside of the Leg

Sen Line – Sahatsarangsi/Thawari, Ittha/Pingkala, Kalathari.

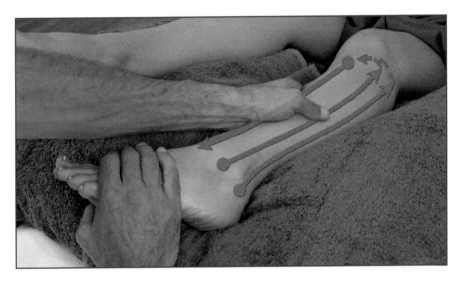

How to...

- Turn the foot towards the midline and hold the foot with your right hand.

- Using the thumb of your left hand just under the lateral ankle. Thumb slide up Sen Ittha/Pingkala, behind the ankle and along below the fibula to the top of the fibula. As you Thumb slide up this line rock forwards.

- At the top of this line slide the thumb medially to the lateral edge of the tibia and slide down Sen Sahatsarangsi/Thawari, along the lateral edge of the tibia to the hollow at the top of the foot. As you thumb

Working the Sen Lines of the Leg

slide down this line rock backwards. Do not try to press with any force as you slide down this line.

- Now thumb slide up Sen Kalathari. Place the thumb of your left hand just above the lateral ankle and then thumb slide up the lower leg just above the fibula, to the top of the fibula. Rock forwards as you slide up this line and then rock backwards as you slide down Sen Sahatsarangsi/Thawari as before.

- Repeat this technique of sliding up Sen Ittha/Pingkla, down Sahatsarangsi/Thawari, up Sen Kalathari and back down Sen Sahatsarangsi/Thawari between three to five times.

- Then thumb slide with alternate thumbs up along Sen Sahatsarangsi/Thawari, from the hollow at the top of the foot, along the lateral edge of the tibia, to the top of the tibia.

81 ~ Thumb Slide the Sen Lines on the Inside of the Leg

Sen Line – Sahatsarangsi/Thawari, Kalathari.

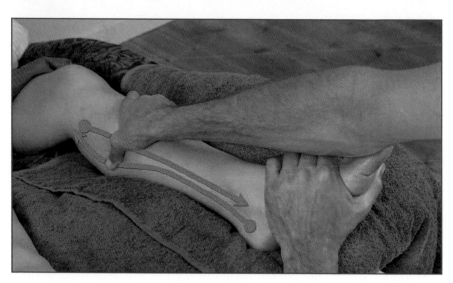

How to...

- Turn the foot laterally and hold the foot in your left hand.

- Using your right thumb, thumb slide up the inside of the lower leg along Sen Kalathari. Starting between the medial ankle and the Achilles tendon, up over the medial head of the calf muscle.

Working the Sen Lines of the Leg

- Then slide the thumb laterally slightly, and slide the thumb down Sen Sahatsarangsi/Thawari on the inside of the leg.

- Rock forwards as you thumb slide up Sen Kalathari and backwards as you slide down Sen Sahatsarangsi/Thawari. Repeat this three to five times.

- Then thumb slide with alternate thumbs up along Sen Sahatsarangsi/Thawari from just behind the medial ankle along the medial edge of the tibia to the top of the tibia.

Percussions on the Legs and Feet

82 ~ Stroke Off the Calf and Achilles

Sen Line – Sumana.

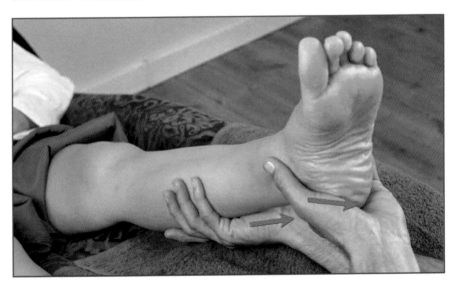

How to...

- Reach with your right hand, halfway along the lower leg.

- Hold the back of the lower leg in your right hand and stroke in one movement down the lower leg and off the heel.

- Now repeat with your left hand.

Working the Sen Lines of the Leg

- You should feel warmth on the back of the leg as you do this.

- Repeat this 10 times.

- This technique can also be performed standing up so that the leg is lifted off the couch.

- If you perform the technique standing up you will drop the leg into the ready and waiting other hand as you stroke off the heel.

- As you catch the leg in your other hand you can "cup" the leg by meeting the leg with a cupped hand and gentle slap.

- This technique takes a little practice, but becomes quicker and more fluid.

83 ~ Pummel the Back of the Lower Leg

Sen Line – Sumana.

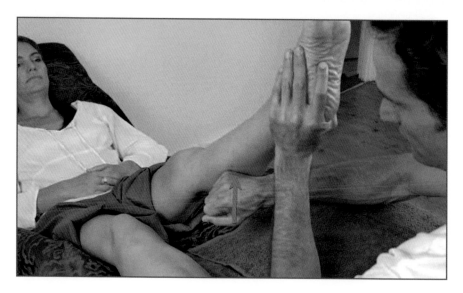

How to...

- If you were standing for the last move sit back down.

- Rest your left elbow on the couch, so that your left palm is facing upwards, rather like a waiter holding a tray.

Working the Sen Lines of the Leg

- Support the foot in this left hand so that the leg is lifted off of the couch.

- Make a loose fist with your right hand and pummel the back of the leg with the little finger edge of your loose fist

- Work all around the back of the lower leg with this technique.

84 ~ Pummel the Sole of the Foot

Sen Line – Kalathari.

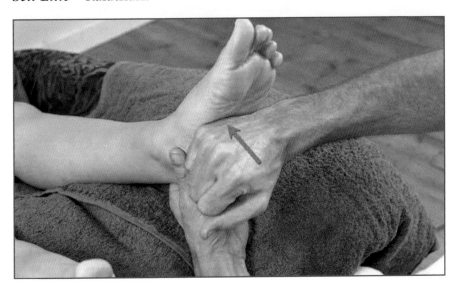

How to...

- Bring the leg back down to rest on the couch and whilst still supporting the foot in your left hand pummel or backhand (as before) the sole of the foot.

- Restrict this move to the sole of the foot, between the heel and the balls of the toes.

85 ~ Pummel the Outside of the Leg

Sen Line – Sahatsarangsi/Thawari, Ittha/Pingkala, Kalathari.

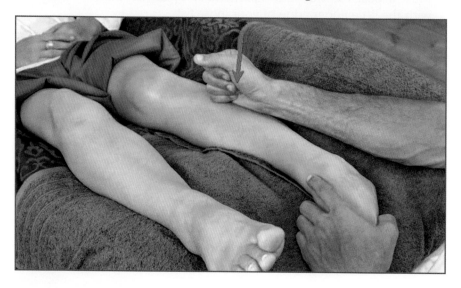

How to...

- Turn the foot towards the midline and hold the foot with your left hand.
- Make a loose fist with your right hand and pummel the outside of the lower leg between the tibia and fibula.
- Work up and then back down making sure that you stay between the 2 bones, and not on them.
- Repeat 3 times.

86 ~ Pummel the Inside of the Leg

Sen Line – Kalathari, Sahatsarangsi/Thawari.

How to...

- Turn the foot laterally and hold the foot with your right hand.
- Make a loose fist with your left hand and pummel the inside of the lower leg below the Tibia.

Working the Sen Lines of the Leg

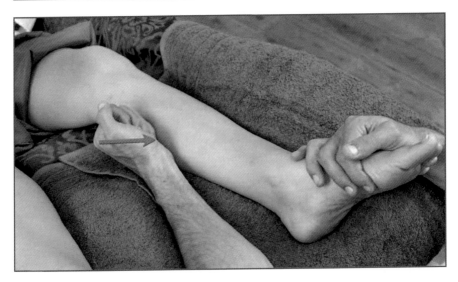

- Work up and then back down making sure that you stay below the Tibia.

- Repeat 3 times.

87 ~ Thumb Circle the Ankle

Sen Line – Ittha/Pingkala, Sahatsarangsi/Thawari.

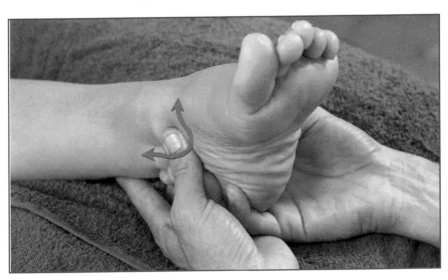

How to…

- Place the fingers of both hands underneath the Achilles tendon and heel of the foot and rest your right thumb on the outside of the ankle and your left thumb on the inside of the ankle.

- Now work the thumbs in a half moon shape around the inside and outside of the ankle.

- Start near to the hollow at the front of the foot with both thumbs. The right thumb near to the lateral edge and the left thumb near to the medial edge.

- Slide the thumbs apart so that they stroke down next to the front of the medial and lateral ankle as you rock your body backwards.

- Then slide the thumbs up behind the medial and lateral ankle as you rock your body forwards.

- Now slide back down behind the ankle and then back up to near the hollow.

- Repeat this 10 times, remembering to rock your body as you move your thumbs.

Wrapping the Feet

88 ~ Wrap the Foot and the Leg

Sen Line – Sumana, Kalathari, Ittha/Pingkala, Sahatsarangsi/Thawari.

How to…

- It now becomes important that the towels were set up correctly at the start.

- Make sure that the leg is resting down the centre line of the towel, and that the top of the towel is level with the top of the lower leg near to the knee.

- This should give you some free towel to wrap the foot with.

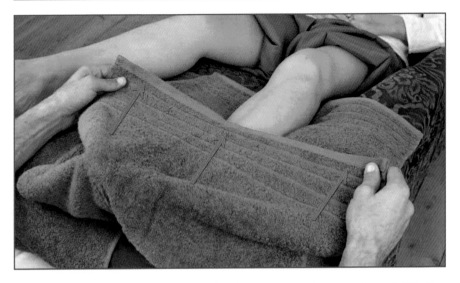

Step 1: Hold the 2 corners of the bottom of the towel and lift the towel so that the towel is flat against the sole of the foot.

Step 2: Drape the bottom of the towel over the toes onto the top of the foot or the leg (depending on the leg length).

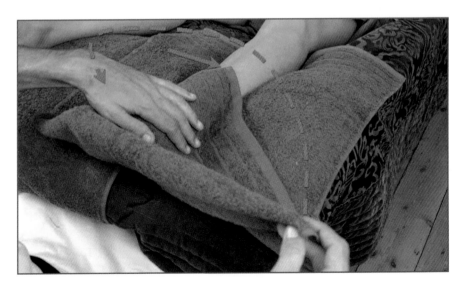

Step 3: Bring the medial corner of the towel to the lateral edge of the tibia, and hold the towel flat against the top of the foot with your left hand.

Working the Sen Lines of the Leg

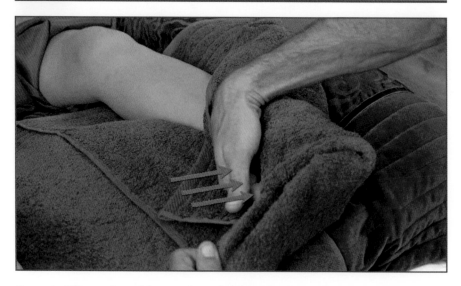

Step 4: There should now be a fold at the lateral edge of the towel. Hold the corner of this fold with your right hand, and fold the lateral edge of the towel back over the top of the foot and tuck it between the medial edge of the towel and the medial fold of the towel so it tucks back under the medial arch of the foot.

Step 5: Pull gently with your left hand on the medial edge of the towel as you tuck the towel further under the medial arch of the foot. This should wrap the foot quite tightly.

Now wrap the leg.

Step 1: Hold the medial edge of towel with both hands, your right hand about midway along the edge and your left hand near to the top of the towel at the knee.

Step 2: Draw the medial edge of the towel further towards the midline so that there is hardly any towel left showing laterally, and there is enough towel showing medially to wrap around the whole leg.

Be careful not to pull the towel down, keep it long so that there is still towel near to the knee

Step 3: Bring the medial edge of the towel over the leg and the top of the foot.

Working the Sen Lines of the Leg

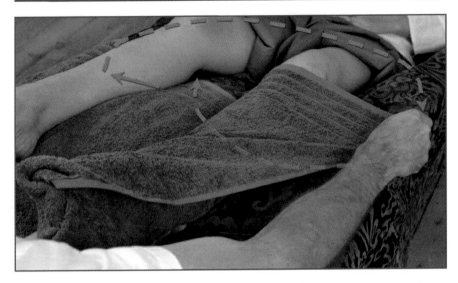

Step 4: Try to keep the towel tight against the leg as you continue to bring the edge of the towel back under the lower leg and return it to the medial side of the lower leg.

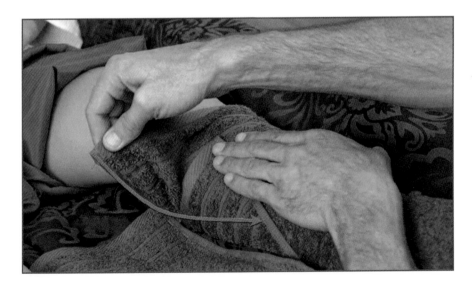

Step 5: Pull the corner of the towel to tighten the towel around the leg.

Step 6: Fold the top of the towel down over this corner to hold the towel in place.

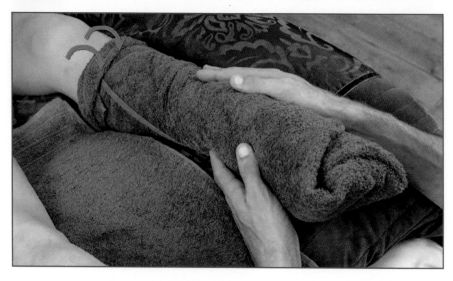

Now unwrap the towel and try again! This takes a few goes to get the hang of, but it feels great when the towel is wrapped nice and tightly.

Now repeat for other leg from the Opening Sequence.

When you have completed the first three sections on both legs continue onto the closing section.

The Closing Sequence

Both legs should now be wrapped up having been thoroughly massaged. This section is the beginning of the end of the massage. It begins by working the legs through the wraps and involves some gentle stretches that continue to open the Sen lines whilst also awakening your partner.

Working Through the Wraps

Working through the wraps gives an entirely different feeling to the massage. The techniques are all presses as opposed to sliding techniques and give a feeling similar to a Traditional Thai Massage. The emphasis is on working the Sen Lines here, however Reflex points are also worked, but much more generally.

  The techniques are similar to previous techniques, but it is much harder to be sure where you are working when working through the wraps so pay attention to the landmarks such as the bones as these will be easier to feel through the wraps.

89 ~ Thumb Press the Centre Line on the Sole of the Foot

Sen Line – Sahatsarangsi/Thawari, Kalathari.
Reflex Points – Sexual organs, insomnia point, sigmoid colon (left foot), small intestines, transverse colon, kidney, solar plexus, lung.

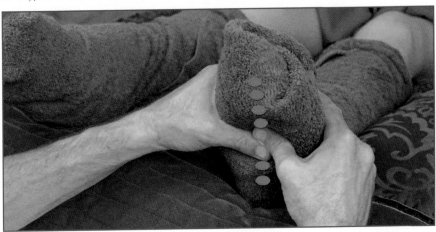

How to...

- Place both thumbs, one above the other at the centre of the heel on the bottom of the foot.

- Gently rest your fingers on the dorsum of the foot.

- Rock forwards as you thumb press into the heel with both thumbs, and rock backwards as you release.

- Move the thumbs slightly higher and continue up to the ball of the centre toe

- Repeat coming back down the centre line of the foot.

Intention

Sahatsarangsi/Thawari is touched on here to assist the function of the knee joint. The main work is on Sen Kalathari and the reflex points it covers. The intention here is a last push of energy from the feet up through the body.

90 ~ Thumb Press Sen Kalathari on Top of the Foot

Sen Line – Kalathari.

Reflex Points – Lymph nodes (chest), chest, labyrinth (inner ear), ribs, diaphragm, larynx trachea and vocal chords, hip joint.

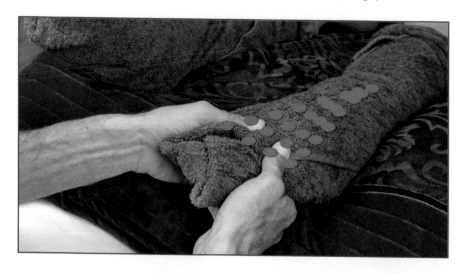

The Closing Sequence

How to...

- Hold the foot in both hands with your thumbs on the top of the foot and your fingers on the sole of the foot.
- Starting in the channels between the first knuckle of the toes. Thumb press along 2 of the channels between the metatarsals of the foot to the depression or hollow in front of the ankle, and then back to between the first knuckle of the toes. Thumb press 2 channels at a time.
- Now repeat for the next 2 channels.
- The fifth channel runs from lateral edge of the little toe to the hollow in front of the ankle. Thumb press this channel from the toe up to the hollow and then back to the toe.

Intention

The working of Sen Kalathari in this and the two following techniques is intended to steady your client emotionally and physically steady the heartbeat and breathing, whilst encouraging the energy flow up through the body.

91 ~ Thumb Press the Sen Kalathari on the Outside of the Leg

Sen Line – Kalathari.

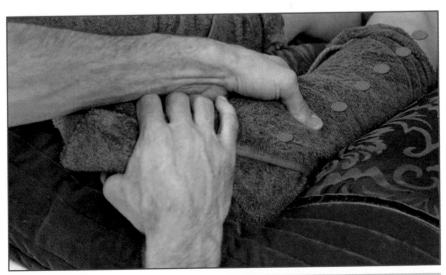

How to...

- Turn the foot towards the midline and hold with your right hand.

- Using the thumb of your left hand, thumb press up Sen Kalathari. Place the thumb of your left hand just above the lateral ankle and then thumb press up the lower leg just above the fibula, to the top of the fibula and then back down. Each time you thumb press along this line rock forwards. Press at 5 or 6 points along this line.

92 ~ Thumb Press Sen Kalathari on the Inside of the Leg

Sen Line – Kalathari.

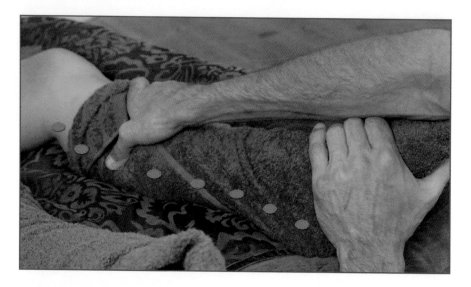

How to...

- Turn the foot laterally and hold in your left hand.

- Using your right thumb, thumb press up and then back down the inside of the lower leg along the Sen Kalathari. Starting between the medial ankle and the Achilles tendon, up over the medial head of the calf muscle.

- Rock forwards each time you thumb press.

93 ~ Rotate the Foot

Sen Line – Sumana, Kalathari, Ittha/Pingkala, Sahatsarangsi/ Thawari (none directly).

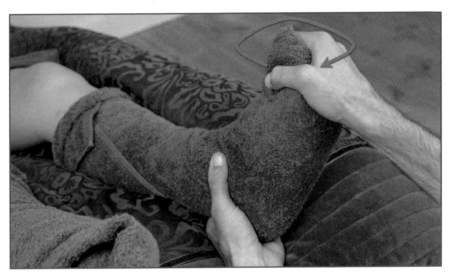

How to...

- Hold the foot in your right hand so that the heel of your hand is against the balls of the toes and the fingers are over the toes touching the top of the foot.
- Support the heel of the foot with your left hand.
- Rotate the foot using the entire range of movement at the ankle joint, 5 times one way and then 5 times the other way.
- It feels nice with this move if you hold the toes tightly in your hands.

Intention

To open all of the Sen Lines running through the ankle joint.

94 ~ Twist the Foot and Stretch the Leg Laterally

Sen Line – all but not directly.

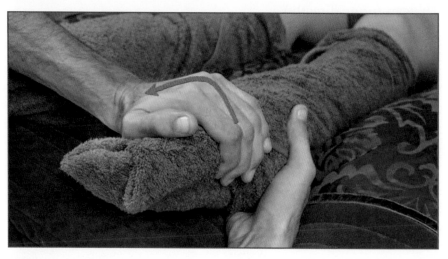

How to...

- Continue supporting the heel in your left hand.

- With your right hand reach around the top of the foot from the lateral edge to the medial arch, so that your fingers can grasp the medial arch and your hand covers the top of the foot.

- Starting nearest the ankle, bend your wrist so that it presses the lateral edge of the foot medially and your fingers pull the medial arch of the foot laterally. Rock backwards as you do this and gently stretch the whole leg.

- Lean forwards as you release the stretch, move your hand further up the top of the foot towards the toes and repeat the stretch as you lean backwards.

- Now move your hand back down and repeat the stretch from the first position.

- Repeat this sequence three times.

Intention

To open the Sen lines on the inside of the leg, by mobilising the joints of the ankle, knee and hip.

The Closing Sequence

95 ~ Twist the Foot and Stretch the Leg Medially

Sen Line – all but not directly.

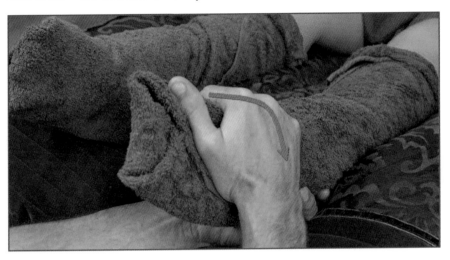

How to...

- Now support the heel in your right hand.

- With your left hand reach around the top of the foot from the medial arch to the lateral edge, so that your fingers can grasp the lateral edge and your hand covers the top of the foot.

- Starting nearest the ankle, bend your wrist so that it presses the medial arch of the foot laterally and your fingers pull the lateral edge of the foot medially. Rock backwards as you do this and gently stretch the whole leg.

- Lean forwards as you release the stretch, move your hand further up the top of the foot towards the toes, and repeat the stretch as you lean backwards.

- Now move your hand back down and repeat the stretch from the first position.

- Repeat this sequence three times.

Intention

To open the Sen lines on the outside of the leg, by mobilising the joints of the ankle, knee and hip.

The Closing Sequence

96 ~ Unwrap the Foot and Drape the Towel over the Leg

How to…

- To unwrap the leg and foot, start by unfolding the top of the towel and then as you continue to unwrap the towel wipe the towel down the leg and foot to remove any remaining cream.

- Then drape the towel over the foot. Do not fold the towel just drape it to cover the foot and as much of the leg that it will cover.

Intention

To remove any remaining excess oil on the leg and foot.

Repeat from 89 on the other leg and then continue on to number 97 where you will work both feet together

Stretching the Feet

This section continues with some more stretches performed on both legs at the same time, which are intended to mobilise the joints and elongate muscles to open the energy lines through the joints and soft tissues.

97 ~ Press the Toes Up

Sen Line – all but not directly.

How to…

- Hold the left foot in your right hand with the heel of the hand against the balls of the toes and the fingers over the toes touching the top of the foot.

- Hold the right foot in the same way with your left hand.

- Press the balls of the foot in the direction of the legs by leaning forwards with your body.

The Closing Sequence

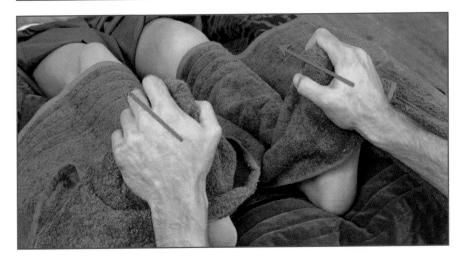

- Hold the stretch briefly and then release the stretch as you lean backwards. Keep holding onto the feet.

- Repeat this stretch 3 times.

Intention

This stretch specifically opens Sen Sumana along the back of the legs, and also Sen Ittha/Pingkala behind the Fibula.

98 ~ Press the Toes Down

Sen Line – all but not directly.

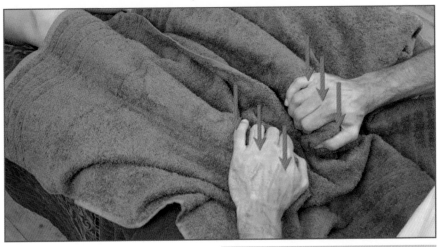

The Closing Sequence

How to...

- Place your hands on the top of the feet, right hand on left foot and left hand on right foot.

- Start with the hands at the top of the dorsum near to where the foot joins the leg.

- Press the feet downwards causing the feet to plantar flex by leaning forwards.

- Release this stretch by leaning backwards.

- Move your hands down the dorsum of the foot to the middle of the dorsum and repeat the stretch.

- Move your hands down to near to the toes and repeat the stretch.

- Now move your hands back up to the middle of the dorsum and repeat the stretch and again at the starting point.

Intention

This stretch specifically opens Sen Sahatsarangsi/Thawari and Sen Kalathari.

99 ~ Cross Stretch the Feet

Sen Line – all but not directly.

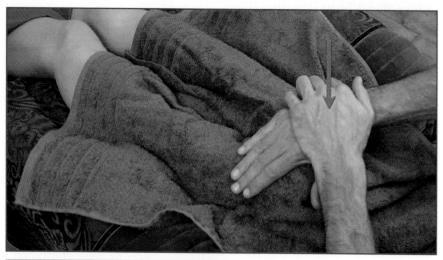

The Closing Sequence

How to...

- Press the left foot medially as far as it will comfortably go and hold it there.

- Press the right medially as well so that the medial arch of the right foot rests on the dorsum of the left foot.

- Hold the right foot with both hands so that the left foot stays where it is.

- Press down gently 3 times creating a stretch along the lateral ankle and lateral lower leg.

- Uncross the feet and then again cross the feet in the same manner with right foot under the left foot this time, and gently press 3 times.

Intention

This stretch is specific to Sen Kalathari on the outside of the leg.

100 ~ Pull the Toes

Sen Line – Kalathari.

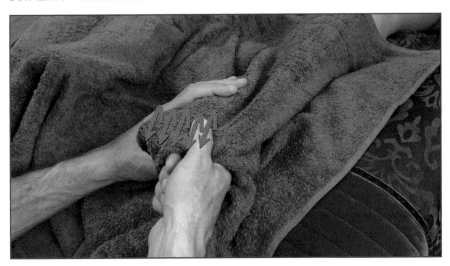

How to...

- Starting with the little toe of the left foot and working along the toes to the little toe of the right foot.

The Closing Sequence

- Hold the toe near to the base of the toe between thumb and first finger, again, as if you were passing a card to someone.

- Gently lift the toe upwards, which may lift the entire foot slightly.

- If there is a popping sound in one or more of the joints of the toe lower the foot.

- If there is no popping sound, continue to gently but firmly pull the toe towards you and then place the foot back down.

- Whether there is a popping sound or not continue to the next toe and repeat this movement once for each toe.

NB: If you or your partner find this popping sensation uncomfortable either skip this technique or replace with a more gentle stretch of each toe.

Intention

To stretch the toes and release energy through the joints of the toes.

Awakening the Feet and Legs

This section begins with some techniques on and above the knees to encourage the energy further up the body, and then moves back down to the foot for some brisk techniques to awaken the feet and legs, and maybe your partner.

101 ~ Warm Your Hands and Cover the Knees

Sen Line – Sahatsarangsi/Thawari.

How to...

- Place your hands together in the welcoming posture and then gently rub the hands together in a circular motion creating a lot of heat in the hands.

The Closing Sequence

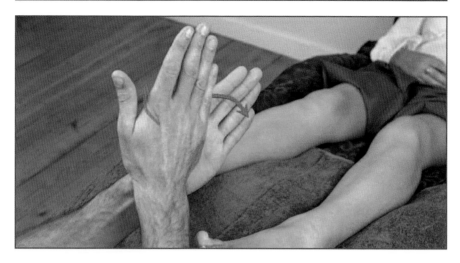

- Now place your hands gently on the knees. The right hand on the left knee and the left hand on the right knee.

- This warmth on the knees feels great on an area of the body that lacks in circulation.

Intention

To warm the knee and encourage energy to flow past the knee.

102 ~ Palm Circle the Knees

Sen Line – Sahatsarangsi/Thawari.

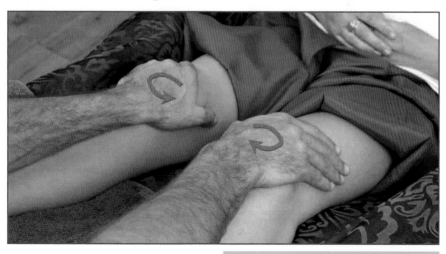

The Closing Sequence

How to...

- Keep your hands on the knees and gently circle your hands on the knees so that you press gently up and then out and back down.

Intention

To warm the knee further and encourage energy to flow around and past the knee.

---

103 ~ Thumb Press 3 Points on the Thigh

Sen Line – Sahatsarangsi/Thawari.

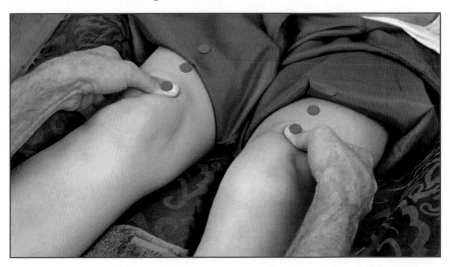

How to...

- Place your thumbs on the centre line of the thigh, just above the knee, so that the right thumb is on the left leg and the left thumb is on the right leg. Your fingers should be resting gently on the outside of the thighs.

- Lean forwards and press with the pads of the thumbs into the thighs.

- Move your thumb up 1 thumb length along the centre line and thumb press again.

- Move your thumb up another thumb length and press for a third time.

- Move your thumbs back down and press again on the second point and then down again to the first point.

Intention

To encourage energy flow from the knee upwards.

104 ~ Finger Circle Behind the Knees

Sen Line – Sumana.

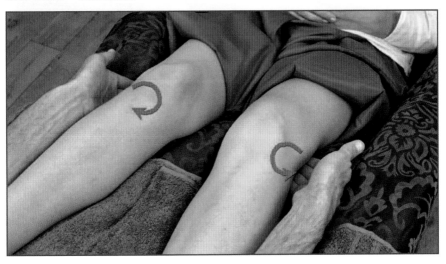

How to...

- Slide your fingers under the back of the knees and circle the skin there.

- Using all of the fingers gently press against the soft skin there and circle the fingers of both hands down and towards you and then out and up.

- As you circle the hands don't let the fingers slide over the skin, instead move the skin with the fingertips.

- Repeat this circle 5–10 times.

Intention

This technique assists with Lymphatic drainage in the Popliteal area behind the knee and encourages the energy to flow past the knee.

105 ~ Palm Press the Outside of the Lower Leg

Sen Line – Kalathari, Sahatsarangsi/Thawari.

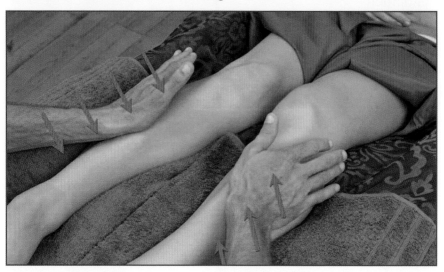

How to...

- Use the heel of your hands to press down the lateral edge of both legs.

- Place the heel of the hands at the top of the lower leg, along the lateral edge of the leg, between the lateral edge of the tibia and the fibula.

- Press with the heel of the hand by bending at the wrist as you press along the lateral edge of the leg.

- Move down the leg towards the ankle and repeat the press.

- Continue all the way down to the bottom of the lower leg.

Intention

The last technique before returning to the feet, and the last push of energy along the Sen Lines of the legs.

106 ~ Thumb Circle the Outside and Inside of the Ankle

Sen Line – Kalathari and Ittha/Pingkala (laterally) Sahatsarangsi/ Thawari (medially).

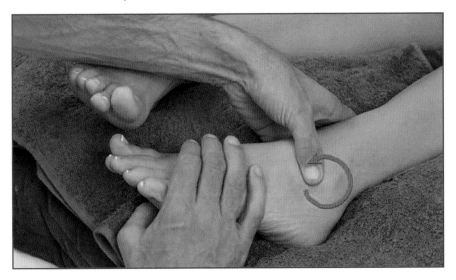

How to...

- Turn the left foot medially and hold it with your right hand.
- Use the thumb of your left hand to circle around the lateral ankle. The fingers of your left hand should be resting on the foot and pointing towards or on the medial ankle.
- Circle the thumb all the way around the ankle about 10 times.
- This technique is quite brisk and does not need much pressure.
- Now turn the foot laterally and hold with your left hand.
- Use your right hand to circle the medial ankle.

Intention

This brisk technique begins to warms and re awaken the foot.

107 ~ Thumb Slide the Medial Arch of the Foot

Sen Line – Sumana.
Reflex Points – Spine.

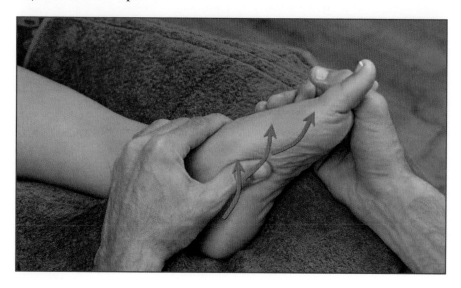

How to...

- Place your left thumb near the heel along the medial arch of the foot and slide the thumb along the medial arch.

- Use a slight flicking motion so that the thumb slides off of the medial arch, and then move the thumb up along the medial arch slightly nearer the toes and repeat the flicking motion.

- Continue along the medial arch of the foot and repeat 3 times.

Intention

A stimulating technique to awaken the foot and the spine, and to send energy from the foot up through the body.

108 ~ Thumb Stroke and Stretch the Toes

Sen Line – Kalathari.

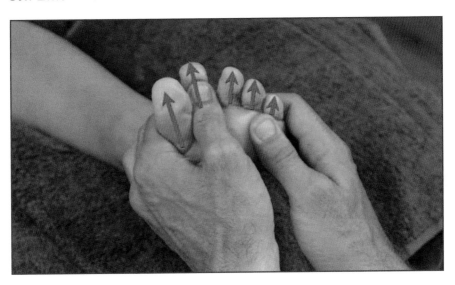

How to...

• Bring the foot back to the centre position and use the thumb of both hands to stroke the toes back.

• If you start with your right thumb gently stroke one of the toes away from you so that the toe gets a gentle stretch and stroke.

• As you stroke off the toe with your right thumb, begin on another toe with your left thumb, and repeat until all the toes have been gently stretched and stroked a few times.

Intention

A gentle stretch of each toe which encourages the flow of energy and circulation to the extremities and begins to awaken the senses and the brain.

109 ~ Slap and Stroke the Dorsum of the Foot

Sen Line – Kalathari.

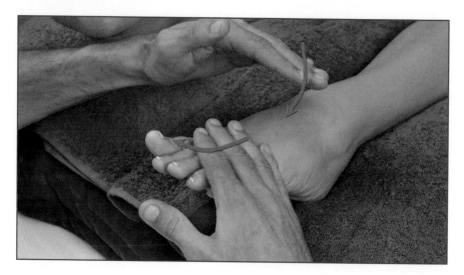

How to...

- Using all the fingers of both hands slap and stroke the dorsum of the foot in a circular motion.

- Place the fingers of your right hand on the dorsum of the foot, and stroke off the toes towards you.

- As your right hand strokes off the toes, gently slap the top of the foot with your left hand, and then stroke off the foot towards the toes with your left hand.

- As your left hand strokes off the toes, your right hand gently slaps the top of the foot and continues to stroke off the foot.

- Continue this circular motion.

- This is a very brisk technique when you get the hang of it.

Intention

A very stimulating technique to awaken your partner!

Now repeat 106–109 on the other foot before
finishing the massage with 110.

The Closing Sequence

110 ~ Cup the Outside of Both Legs

Sen Line – Kalathari, Sahatsarangsi/Thawari.

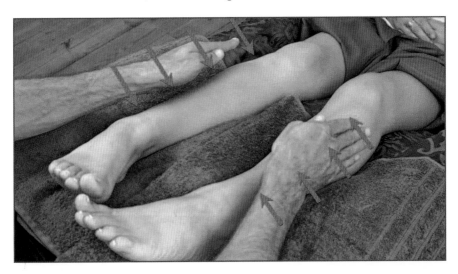

How to...

- Place your hands in the welcome or prayer position, but open the palms of the hands slightly, so that the fingertips and thumbs are still together, as well as the heel of the hand, but there is now space between the hands.

- If you move your hands apart now and then clap them together you should hear a cupping sound as opposed to a clapping sound.

- Starting near to the ankle on the lateral edge of both the lower legs, between the tibia and fibula.

- Cup up and down the lateral edge of both legs simultaneously.

- Try to make this more of a cup than a slap.

- Bring your hands together in respect for your client and to signify the end of the massage.

Intention

This last technique encourages the flow of energy up through the body and also makes sure your partner is awake.

To Finish...

A Thai Foot Massage will always end as it began, with your hands together in the prayer position, but unlike the prayer at the start of the massage which is performed in honour of Doctor Jivaka Khumarabhacca, this prayer is directed at your partner. Often no words are said, but you may repeat the last line of the Traditional prayer.

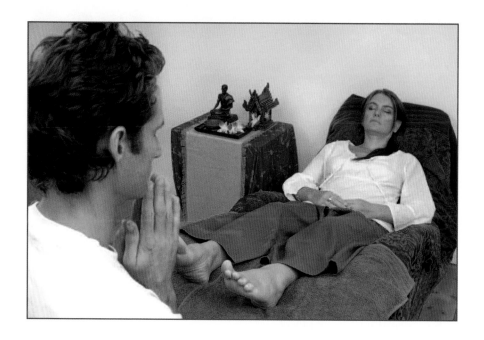

Na-A Na-Wa Rokha Payati Vina-Santi

We pray for the one whom we touch,
that they will be happy
and that any illness will be released from them.

It is important to give your partner time to relax after a massage. If you are using a recliner chair allow them to rest in the chair for a few minutes before bringing the chair into an upright position. Allow your partner time to rest in the upright position for few more minutes and bring them something to drink, either a herbal tea, or water is customary.

This may or may not be an appropriate time to get some feedback, but at least try to arrange their next massage before parting.

Some Notes on Shortening the Massage

The Thai Foot Massage sequence that you have just practised is very comprehensive and includes all of the techniques. At some point you will probably want to shorten the treatment, and it is up to you how you do this, however I have some suggestions that may help.

For a one hour treatment, complete all four sections, leaving out a few techniques from each section, but try to work all of the points with the stick.

For a treatment of half an hour or less, leave out the stick section completely and perform just a few techniques from the closing sequence.

Bibliography

Apfelbaum, Ananda. *Thai Massage: Sacred Bodywork*. New York: Avery, 2004

Brust, Harald (Asokananda). *The Art of Traditional Thai Massage*. Bangkok: Editions Duang Kamol, 1990

Brust, Harald (Asokananda) and Chow Kam Thye. *The Art of Traditional Thai Massage Energy Line Charts*. Bangkok: Editions Duang Kamol, 1995

Chokevivat, Vichai and Anchalee Chuthaputti. *The Role of Thai Traditional Medicine in Health Promotion*. Bangkok: Department for the Development of Thai Traditional and Alternative Medicine, Ministry of Public Health, Thailand, 2005

Frawley, David, Subhash Ranade and Avinash Lele. *Ayurveda and Marma Therapy: Energy Points in Yogic Healing*. Twin Lakes, WI: Lotus Press, 2003

Issel, Christine. *Reflexology: Art, Science & History*. Sacramento, CA: New Frontier Publishing, 1990

Salguero, C. Pierce. *Encyclopedia of Thai Massage*. Findhorn, Scotland: Findhorn Press, 2004

Salguero, C. Pierce. *Thai Massage Workbook*. Findhorn, Scotland: Findhorn Press, 2007

Setthakorn, Chongkol. *Ancient Massage of Thailand*. Chiang Mai, Thailand: Sang Ngern Printing, 1992

Wilson, Tananan. *Nerve Touch Massage*. Chiang Mai, Thailand, 2003

Resources

For professional training in Thai Foot Massage with Simon Piers Gall, and other forms of Traditional Massage contact:

> The London School of Traditional Massage
> www.lstm.com
> info@lstm.com

To find a practitioner near you contact the Association of Thai Massage Therapists:

> www.atmt.org
> info@atmt.org

Matt Gall, cover designer:

> Web design to garden design contact:
> www.thirdwavemusic.com
> info@thirdwavemusic.com

Nick ffrench, photographer:

> Professional photographic services:
> www.nickffrenchphotos.co.uk

Related titles from Findhorn Press by C. Pierce Salguero:

> *A Thai Herbal*
> *Encyclopedia of Thai Massage*
> *Thai Massage Workbook*
> *The Spiritual Healing of Traditional Thailand*

About The Author

Simon Gall is a holistic therapist and teacher of Traditional Thai Massage, in all its many aspects. Following an inspirational study trip to Thailand he founded the London School of Traditional Massage (previously the London School of Thai Massage) in order to promote Thai Massage in the UK.

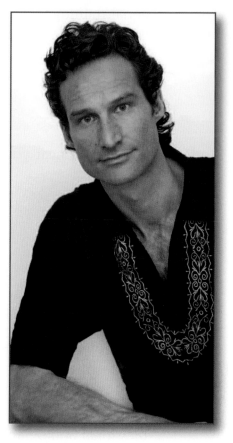

Simon now teaches internationally, to interested therapists and has also helped many Western spas integrate Traditional Thai Massage into their treatments.

He has trained throughout Thailand, at many schools and with many teachers, and learnt Traditional Thai Massage from some of the few remaining Masters of this practice.

Simon is also a trained yoga teacher and specialises in the Traditional Thai form, known as Thai Yogha or Ruesi Dutton.

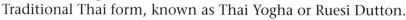

When Simon is not travelling or studying he teaches and practices from The Paula Lloyd Therapy Centre in SE London and from his home in Kent.